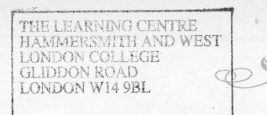
Brown Skin is a treasure trove of
information and advice . . .

Part One: Your Beauty Basics

What makes skin of color different? . . . What is your skin type? Daily skin care
routines . . . The sun and your skin: what you must know . . . Matching makeup
to your skin tone . . . Easy camouflage tips . . . Avoiding common makeup mistakes
. . . Your makeup tool kit . . . Relaxed hair—how many touch-ups? . . . Hints for
hot-combed hair . . . Knockout natural hair, from Afros to weaves . . . Must-have
hair tools . . . Nail dos and don'ts . . . The perfect at-home manicure . . . The lowdown on high-tech: acids, peels, lasers, and more . . . Winning against wrinkles . . .
The lifestyle your skin will love . . . *and more.*

Part Two: Top Skin-of-Color Concerns

Dark marks, blemishes, spots, and patches . . . Allergic reactions . . . Cold sores . . .
Nail fungus . . . Stretch marks . . . Torn earlobes . . . Vitiligo . . . Will cocoa butter
lighten dark marks? . . . Do foods cause acne breakouts? . . . Care for acne-prone skin
. . . Eczema skin care . . . Scar-prevention strategies . . . Coping with keloids . . .
and more.

Part Three: Total Beauty for Life

The changes of pregnancy . . . Great skin, hair, and nails at any age . . . What to
do about hair loss . . . Quiz: Are you harming your hair? . . . All about hair removal
. . . Age-defying solutions for mature women of color . . . Especially for men:
skin-friendly shaving, hair and scalp care, neat nails . . . Skin, hair, and nail TLC
for children of color: babies, toddlers, and teens . . . *and more.*

Amistad

AN IMPRINT OF *HARPERCOLLINS*PUBLISHERS

BROWN SKIN

DR. SUSAN TAYLOR'S

PRESCRIPTION FOR FLAWLESS SKIN, HAIR, AND NAILS

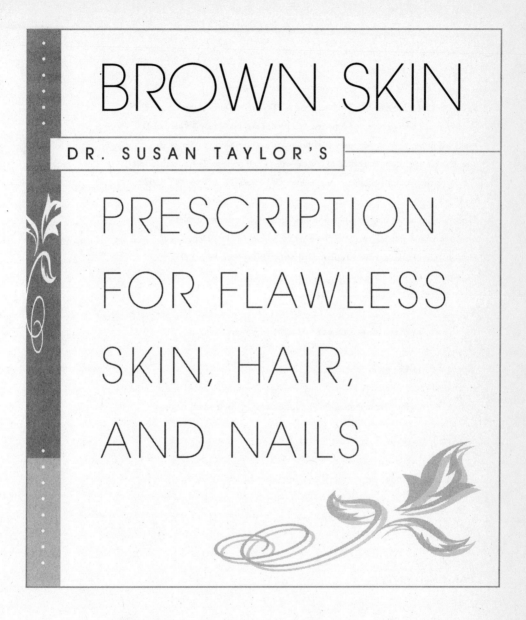

Susan C. Taylor, M.D.

FIRST AMISTAD PAPERBACK EDITION 2004

DESIGNED BY DEBORAH KERNER/DANCING BEARS DESIGN

Printed on acid-free paper

Library of Congress Cataloging-in-Publication Data is available upon request.

ISBN 0-06-008872-9

04 05 06 07 08 BVG/RRD 10 9 8 7 6 5 4 3 2 1

To my family, whose love nurtures, sustains, and propels me forward.

First and foremost my mother, Ethel Hendricks Taylor;
my father, Charles Taylor;
my sister, Flora Taylor;
my husband, Kemel Dawkins,
and my daughters, Morgan and Madison Dawkins.

ACKNOWLEDGMENTS

To my agents, Madeleine Morel and Barbara Lowenstein at Lowenstein-Morel Associates, for their commitment to this project.

To my editor, Toni Sciarra, and the wonderful staff at HarperCollins Publishers for working to bring this much-needed book to fruition.

To Ziba Kashef, whose research and writing assistance have been invaluable.

To Chanelle Harville, Nzingha, Cynde Watson, and Netara Love for their expertise and guidance with the art of makeup.

To Vincent DeLeo, M.D., for believing in the Skin of Color Center.

CONTENTS

311732

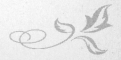

BEFORE YOU
BEGIN THIS BOOK

We all want to look our best, to make the most of our natural beauty. As women of color, we've been blessed with certain advantages, including special skin properties that protect us from the damaging effects of the sun, as well as from the fine and deep wrinkles associated with aging. We also have the benefit of naturally warm, glowing complexions that range in shade from vanilla to cinnamon to deep chocolate brown.

But our special skin is often more reactive and easily damaged by everyday injuries, rashes, and pimples. It is more prone to particular problems, including unsightly discolorations and devastating scars. Even skin conditions common to all skin types can have a completely different, and sometimes disfiguring, appearance on our skin.

While there is no lack of beauty and skin-care information on bookstore shelves these days, few health and beauty books address the unique skin-care needs of women of color. Those that do typically devote only one chapter to our concerns. As a dermatologist and woman of color, I understand how woefully inadequate those chapters often are in educating us about the particular properties of our skin. Written by makeup artists, models, estheticians, and even physicians, these books offer general information and only skim the surface of our needs. This book

provides you with comprehensive and culturally specific how-to information about the skin, hair, and nails of people of color from a woman dermatologist of color.

In this book, I answer the types of questions I frequently hear not only from the various television interviewers, magazine editors, and fellow dermatologists who seek facts about skin of color but also from the many patients I see at the Skin of Color Center at St. Luke's–Roosevelt Hospital in New York, where I serve as the director. At the center, a team of renowned dermatologists and physicians conducts pioneering research on the differences between brown, black, and white skin. We are examining the safety and effectiveness of various medications and cosmetics on pigmented skin. We are experimenting with new technologies, such as state-of-the-art laser technology, to determine whether they are appropriate for skin of color.

I know that as patients, women of color prefer a dermatologist who looks like them. You, the reader of this book, also want advice from a practitioner who understands your culture, who knows what women of color do to care for their skin, hair, and nails—and why. You seek guidance from someone who has firsthand knowledge and experience treating the problems common to your skin. Understandably, you want a skin-care expert who can meet you where you are and empathize with you, as well.

My mission is to teach you what you need to know, as a woman of color, to look better now. Whatever the condition of your skin, nails, and hair, you have in your hands the tools to develop a lifelong beauty regimen and maintenance plan. In these pages, you'll find a comprehensive and culturally specific program for caring for your skin. Filled with practical tips, this program will teach you how to assess your skin's condition, and will provide step-by-step instructions on the proper ways to cleanse, moisturize, and protect it in order to avoid or minimize the dark blemishes and other reactions that often occur on the skin. You'll not only learn about the latest skin advances—from chemical peels to microdermabrasion and laser therapy—but also get the facts on which treatments are safe to use on skin of color. I also guide you in selecting the ideal cosmetics to complement your skin from the outside, and I discuss ways to enhance your beauty from the inside through diet, exercise, and other lifestyle strategies.

Like your personal dermatologist, this book provides patient-tested solutions to your most urgent skin, nail, and hair-care challenges. In detailed chapters, the book addresses the five most prevalent skin-care problems brown women face, in addition to a variety of other skin conditions, including skin cancer, and how to treat them. You'll find tips for the care of aging skin of color. You'll learn the true causes of hair thinning and hair loss in our community—which are not normal consequences of aging, as many believe—and how you can prevent and cope with these common hair-care concerns. And because you are probably the primary caregiver in your family, you also get advice on how to help your mate and your children with the skin-care problems that plague them most. They, too, will look their best.

I know you want to make the most of your natural beauty because when you look good, you feel good and have higher self-esteem. The ultimate goal of this book, and the program and patient case histories contained within it, is to help you be your best.

WHAT IS SKIN OF COLOR?

In this book, I use the term "skin of color" interchangeably with the terms "black skin," "brown skin," "African-American skin," "Hispanic skin," and "pigmented skin." "Skin of color" is defined as skin that contains increased amounts of melanin as compared to white skin. The amount of melanin among different women of color can vary dramatically. Scientists have estimated that people of African descent have some thirty-five different hues or shades of skin tone. If you think about the members of your family and extended family, you'll recognize that there are probably even more shades than that!

Most Brown women in the United States are likely to have descended from African, Native American, Latin, and/or European ancestry. These combinations can produce an endless array of skin tones and hair textures. So the bottom line is that there is no one type of brown skin.

"Skin of color" can also be defined by its tendency to develop certain conditions or disease states. The melanin in our skin is made of specialized cells known as melanocytes. These cells can produce more melanin when stimulated by the sun, medications, or certain medical conditions. In some cases, the cause of an increase or decrease in melanin is not fully understood. Because of the reactive and unpredictable nature of our skin, women of color are more likely to suffer from problems such as dark marks and other skin discolorations (postinflammatory hyperpigmentation and postinflammatory hypopigmentation), keloids (large, raised scars), and vitiligo, among others. Our skin also reacts more severely to common conditions such as acne and eczema. Those specific problems, and others, will be discussed in detail in the middle portion of the book (chapters 7 through 11).

"Skin of color" also refers to certain cultural habits and practices that are unique to people of African descent. These practices have significant impact, both negative and positive, on our skin. For example, the practice of self-medicating skin infections or rashes in not uncommon, especially among older Black women, sometimes with disastrous results. Cultural habits and practices also extend to how we care for our nails and hair. The use of hot combs and chemical hair relaxers to straighten tightly curled hair can lead to hair loss that is not observed in women who don't employ these hair-care practices.

Certain myths about skin conditions also abound in the Black community. For example, you may have heard relatives, particularly from the South, say that a particular type of brown growths commonly found on the face and neck of people of color, sometimes called skin tags, cannot be removed because they'll become cancerous or, worse, cause you to bleed to death! However, these growths (known medically as *dermatosis papulosa nigra*) are actually hereditary and normal, and they can be removed safely by a dermatologist to give your skin a smoother and more youthful appearance. Another example is that while certain dark pinpoint holes in the palms of people of color may be normal, other dark spots or moles on the palms or soles can actually indicate diseases such as syphilis or cancer.

As you see, "skin of color" is not just about more melanin but also a complex mix of physical characteristics and cultural beliefs. Understanding the special character of skin of color will help you better care for your skin, recognize and prevent problems, and seek the best treatment when it's needed.

THE SKIN OF COLOR CENTER

The skin-care program and solutions you'll find in these pages are drawn from my more than fifteen years of experience treating patients of color in private practice. Of the two hundred or so patients I see every week in my office in Philadelphia, the majority are people of color who have seen me either on television or quoted in magazines. Some come by referral simply looking for a doctor who looks like them. Most are women who have been searching for answers to their mild to severe skin-care problems for months, or even years. While in my office, they look very closely at my skin and my hair to make sure I practice what I preach and have useful information and tools to offer them.

To better serve my patients and deepen the scientific understanding of skin of color, in 1998 I became director of the Skin of Color Center at St. Luke's Hospital Center in New York City. When I helped establish the Skin of Color Center, it was the first such center of its kind. As the number of people of color in the United States has steadily grown to 24 percent of the population (Blacks constitute 12 percent, Hispanics 10 percent), the need for medical information and expertise specific to pigmented skin has also grown. At the center—where about 90 percent of patients are of color—a cadre of highly regarded dermatologists are clarifying the differences between skin of color and white skin. This groundbreaking work will soon lead to better treatments for skin of color and greater choices for you and all women of color.

Through the center's work, my work at Society Hill Dermatology (www.societyhilldermatology.com) in Philadelphia, and this book, I hope as a health-care practitioner to make a significant contribution to the science of dermatology. As a Black woman, my desire is to benefit the lives of people of color. To best serve the increasing numbers of patients of color, the field of dermatology will need to broaden its focus to include knowledge about pigmented skin, and develop better technologies and products to treat it. Black and Hispanic women, who suffer disproportionately from a variety of medical problems—many of which affect the skin—will certainly gain from the growing body of information and expertise in skin of color. With knowledge, we'll have the tools to make wiser choices and to improve our looks and our well-being.

While training in the specialty of dermatology at Columbia Presbyterian Medical Center in New York in the late 1980s, I realized that the skin was in fact a window onto the body. If there is an internal problem such as lupus, diabetes, or sarcoidosis—all conditions more prevalent among Brown women than White women—signs often first appear in the skin. On the other hand, skin-specific problems that appear on the surface can have a detrimental impact on women emotionally. I take great pride in work that allows me to help the whole patient, both physically and emotionally.

This book is my gift to you. I hope that in accepting it, you'll start to take the health of your skin, nails, and hair as seriously as I do. In transforming your appearance, you can begin transforming the way you feel about yourself and your life. Through good skin care, many of my patients' lives have changed and even flourished. That is my wish for you. If you need information concerning my dermatology practices and the care that I give, contact www.drsusantaylor.net or www.societyhilldermatology.com.

HOW TO USE THIS BOOK

This book is divided into three major sections. The first offers guidance for evaluating your skin and developing a daily skin-care program, with tips on selecting the best skin-care products and techniques—and improving your lifestyle—in order to give a boost to your skin and appearance. The second section provides specific solutions to common skin diseases and skin-care problems for women of color, including hyperpigmentation, acne, eczema, and keloids, among other challenges. The third section answers questions about pregnancy, aging, and hair loss, and offers advice on beauty for the whole family.

You may be tempted to skip ahead to a section that addresses a problem you're facing now. But I recommend that you review the facts and advice in the first six chapters as well. This will help you to fully understand the nature of your unique skin and not only treat a particular problem but also develop an effective program for your needs. Most women of color have more than one skin, nail, or hair-care concern and even more questions. This book is designed to give you comprehensive answers.

As you read the book, take the time to complete the various quizzes and scan the checklists and bulleted points within the chapters. You may be surprised to learn that you have a different skin type than you thought, or that your risk of sun damage is greater than you believed. You may discover that a mark or mole you were concerned about is completely normal, or that a nagging skin problem actually has a solution.

Once you've read through the book and culled tips that speak to your needs, I encourage you to put your program into action. Good skin is no accident—it takes time and care to cultivate and maintain. Your first step may be a trip to the drugstore or the cosmetics counter to buy better products than the ones you currently use, to add sunscreen to your morning routine, or to finally get that mole checked out. If you need to see a dermatologist, make an appointment for a consultation and ask lots of questions based on your new knowledge about your skin.

However you decide to use the tools and advice in this book, don't procrastinate. As women of color, we too often put off taking care of our needs because we're busy juggling our work and home responsibilities and tending to others. But if you can look and feel better starting today, why wait? Looking your best may be easier—and less expensive—than you think. The rewards of an appearance that reflects you at your best and boosts self-esteem are invaluable.

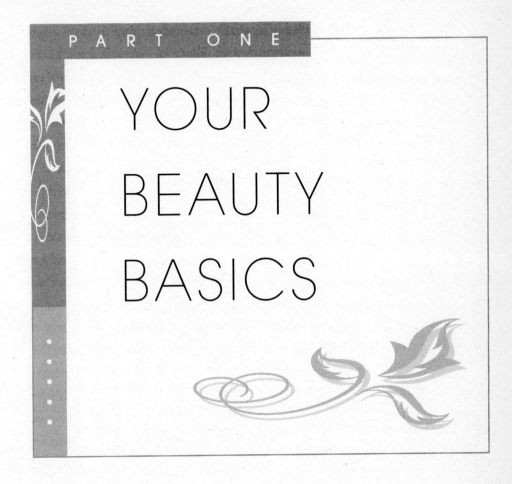

PART ONE

YOUR BEAUTY BASICS

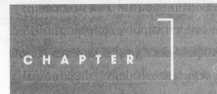

CHAPTER 1

KNOW THY SKIN

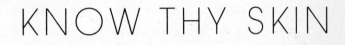

As a woman of color, you've always desired radiant, even-toned skin and healthy, fast-growing hair, but you may not have always had the facts and the guidance you need to look your best. Few books and magazines offer details about the skin and hair of women of color. The books that do offer only superficial, and sometimes inaccurate, information. To get the skin and hair you long for and deserve, you first need to become better acquainted with the skin you're in. As a woman of color, the better you understand what makes your skin and hair unique, the better you'll be able to care for your looks and uncover your natural beauty. In this chapter, you'll begin to learn about skin-of-color characteristics.

Skin of color is quite different from white skin in many respects. Also, among women of color there is great variety of skin tones and types. As you gain a better understanding of the differences between skin of color and white skin, and what makes your skin distinct, you'll be able to make wiser decisions about your skin's care. With this knowledge you'll gain the power to look your best.

In Black and White: What Makes Skin of Color Different?

The distinctions between your skin of color and white skin are numerous. The most notable differences include:

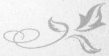

- More melanin, or brown skin pigment, resulting in a warmer skin shade
- Greater natural protection from the sun and lower risk of skin cancer
- Fewer visible signs of aging, such as deep wrinkles, fine lines, and sun spots
- Potential problems with pigmentation, or uneven darkening or lightening of skin
- Greater risk of keloid (raised, often large scars) development

SKIN OF COLOR CHARACTERISTICS

Our skin is made up of three distinct layers: the epidermis, the dermis, and the subcutaneous layer. The only visible layer, the epidermis, is composed mainly of keratinocytes—cells that provide a protective barrier to the skin. The epidermis also contains melanocytes—specialized cells that produce melanin, the brown pigment that gives our skin its rich color. These cells are present in the lowest sublayer of the epidermis, or the basal cell layer (see illustration, page 14). The primary purpose of the melanocyte cell is to make melanin.

Although all people have the same number of melanocyte cells, people of color have melanocytes that are capable of making large amounts of melanin. This increased melanin is what gives skin of color its warm shade. But there is no one type of skin of color. Among individual women of color, the amount of melanin varies dramatically, so that a woman with an abundance of melanin will have deep chocolate-brown skin tone, while a woman with less melanin will have vanilla skin tone. There are numerous shades—an estimated thirty-five shades among women of African descent.

Melanin is not a static substance. That is why our skin changes color in response to various stimuli. Our melanocyte cells can produce more melanin if stimulated by the sun, medications, or certain diseases. The most obvious example of this is tanning, which occurs when our skin produces more melanin after sun exposure. Our skin may also darken in response to certain drugs such as minocycline, which is commonly used to treat acne, or in response to certain medical conditions such as Addison's disease (see "Melanin and Medicine," page 14, and "Melanin and Your Health," page 15). Our skin can also produce less pigmentation, or lightened areas, after a burn or other injury.

The melanin in our skin offers us certain other characteristics that are superior in many respects to white skin. Have you noticed that you look ten years younger than many of your White friends of the same age? This is because of your skin's greater melanin content. Our melanin has many significant health as well as beauty benefits. The most terrific advantage to having large amounts of melanin in the skin is that it protects skin from the damaging impact of the sun. It guards the skin from short-term effects such as severe sunburn (although our skin can burn under certain circumstances). Our melanin also guards our skin from long-term damage associated with aging—the development of deep wrinkles, rough surface texture, and age spots (sometimes called liver spots).

Another advantage to having more melanin is that people of color are less susceptible to developing skin cancer, particularly the more common types known as basal and squamous cell skin cancers. The rate of skin cancer among African Americans, though significant, is many times lower than the rate for Whites. As women of color, we also have the advantage of possessing the naturally warm, glowing skin sought after by White women without having to go to the beach or a tanning salon.

However, we must accept the down sides as well. A disadvantage to having more melanin is that it makes our skin more "reactive." That means almost any stimulus—a rash, scratch, pimple, or inflammation—may trigger the production of excess melanin, resulting in dark marks or patches on the skin. These dark areas are the result of what is called *postinflammatory hyperpigmentation*. Less commonly, some Black women will develop a decrease in melanin or *postinflammatory hypopigmenta-*

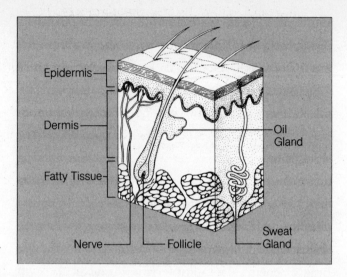

Layers of the skin

Used by permission of the National Cancer Institute [NCI]

tion in response to skin trauma (burns, etc.). In either case, the dark or light areas may be disfiguring and devastating for women who experience them, especially because the discolorations may take months or years to fade. That's why handling your skin gently, wearing sunscreen, and preventing pigmentation problems are keys to our skin care.

Skin of color is also more susceptible to developing certain conditions such as keloids, or large, raised scars that grow beyond the original site of injury. We are more likely to be affected by several different types of disfiguring bumps, such as razor bumps or bumps that occur in the back of the scalp called *acne keloidalis nuchae*. I discuss these conditions and others later in the book.

Melanin and Medicine

A variety of common medications can increase your sensitivity to the sun's ultraviolet (UV) rays, triggering an excess production of melanin and uneven darkening of the skin known as hyperpigmentation. If you are taking any of the following drugs, discuss this possible side effect with your doctor. Be sure to apply a sunscreen with SPF 15 to 30 every day:

- Birth control pills
- Antibiotics (tetracycline, minocycline, doxycycline)
- Blood pressure medication (diuretics or water pills)
- Acne medication (Retin-A, Differin, Tazorac, Accutane)
- Antiseizure medication (Dilantin)
- Certain cancer drugs (Cytoxan, Adriamycin, Bleomycin, Methotrexate, Cyclosporin)
- Rheumatoid arthritis drugs (Methotrexate, Cyclosporin)
- Psoriasis medication (Methotrexate)
- Parkinson's medication (Levodopa)
- Sickle cell medication (Hydroxurea)
- Connective tissue disease medication (Cytoxan)

DID YOU KNOW?

Through DNA studies scientists have confirmed that all people in the world originated from one man and one woman in Africa. Presumably these early people had skin of color. That heritage is rich and unique.

Melanin and Your Health

If you have certain medical conditions, your skin of color can become more susceptible to hyperpigmentation (dark marks). These conditions include:

- Addison's Disease
- Carcinoid Syndrome
- Cirrhosis
- Cutaneous Amyloidosis
- Cushing's Syndrome

- Erythema Dyschromicum Perstans
- Human Immunodeficiency Virus—AIDS
- Hyperthyroidism
- Lupus (systemic, discoid, or drug-induced)
- Papillomatosis (confluent and reticulated)
- Pellagra
- Pheochromocytoma
- Phytophotodermatitis
- Scleroderma

ADDITIONAL SKIN OF COLOR CHARACTERISTICS

As you learn more about what makes skin of color different from White skin, and get to know your unique skin better, you may have questions about certain characteristics. There are a number of features that are unique to normal skin of color. As you read about these characteristics below, take a look at your skin to see which, if any, of these features apply. (If you do not have any of these characteristics, that's also normal!)

On Your Arms. Look at your upper arms. You may see a line separating lighter skin on the inside of the arm from the darker skin on the outside. These are known as *Futcher's lines*. They are a normal, inherited aspect of skin of color.

On Your Chest. If the skin on the middle of your chest is lighter in tone than the skin toward the side of the chest, you have what's known as *mid-line hypopigmentation*. This is a normal sign of skin of color.

On Your Hands. Take a good look at your hands. If the creases in the palms are darker than the other palmar skin, you have *palmar crease hyperpigmentation*. Small pinpoint holes in the palms with a dark core are known as *hyperkeratotic palmar pitting*. Finally, look at your nails. If you have dark brown streaks running from the cuticle to the end of the nails, you have *pigmented nail streaks*. (If, however, you have a streak on only one nail, it could be a sign of cancer that must be evaluated by a dermatologist.)

On Your Lips, Gums. Open wide. You may notice darkened gums around your teeth, known as *gingival hyperpigmentation*. This again is normal in individuals with skin of color.

In Black and White: Hair-raising Distinctions

The hair and scalps of people of color are also quite different from that of Whites. Here's what makes your hair unique:

- Curved hair follicle
- Spiral hair shape
- Fewer elastic fibers anchoring hair follicles to dermis
- Greater incidence of *pseudofolliculitis barbae* (razor bumps) in Blacks who shave
- Greater use of potentially harmful chemicals, hot combs, and other products, which may lead to hair and scalp disorders (see chapter 14)

SKIN TYPES

Like many women of color, you may have always believed that you had oily skin. Even some dermatologists believe the myth that most black skin is oily because oil is more visible on a darker skin surface. But, in fact, skin of color comes in all types, and each type has specific characteristics and needs. The major skin types are dry, oily, and normal. A combination of dry and oily types is known as combination skin or T-zone (to indicate the "T" of your forehead and nose where combination skin tends to be oilier). In addition to these types, your skin may be "sensitive" or particularly prone to irritation, redness, or rashes from commonly available skin- or hair-care products—a problem that is prevalent among Black women. Finally, some Black women may have skin that is *hyperpigmenting*. That means that given certain conditions, such as irritation or injury, the skin will form dark marks. These dark marks may develop anywhere on the skin and may require months or years to fade. A common example of hyperpigmenting skin is the formation of a noticeable dark mark that remains after an acne bump disappears and that may take months to fade.

How can you be sure of your skin type? First try the tissue blot test. (You'll need to perform this test several times a year—during spring, summer, fall, and winter—because your skin changes with the seasons.) Here's how to do it: Wash your face with a neutral (not made for a particular skin type) soap or cleanser (such as Neutrogena for normal skin). Rinse with water. Pat dry with a towel just enough to absorb moisture; do not rub. Wait one hour, and then blot your entire face with a large facial tissue. What do you see?

- If you see oil throughout the tissue, you most likely have oily skin.
- If you see oil only in the T-zone (across forehead, down nose and chin), you most likely have combination skin.
- If you see very little oil throughout, you most likely have normal skin.
- If you see no sign of oil at all and your skin is taut, you most likely have dry skin.
- If your skin feels irritated or slightly itchy, you most likely have sensitive skin.
- If your skin has dark marks that have been present for one month or more, you most likely have hyperpigmenting skin.

In addition to using the tissue test, take the following skin-type quiz:

Quiz: *What Is Your Skin Type?*

1. My skin tends to look:

    a. shiny or greasy

    b. shiny in the T-zone

    c. clear; neither shiny nor ashy

    d. ashen, flaky

    e. red and irritated

    f. blotchy or has dark marks

2. In terms of pimples or blackheads, my skin:

    a. frequently develops both

    b. often develops both on my forehead and chin

    c. occasionally develops a pimple

    d. may break out in pimples (especially before my period)

    e. never develops blemishes, but usually exhibits fine rashes after using various products

    f. develops blemishes that always leave dark marks

3. My pores tend to appear:

    a. visible and large

    b. visible and large in certain areas

    c. small, barely noticeable

    d. neither small nor large

    e. noticeable, but not very prominent

    f. I don't even notice my pores because of all of the dark marks

4. I usually need to wash my face:

    a. three or more times a day

    b. two or three times a day

    c. two times a day

     d. once a day

     e. once a day with water only

     f. twice a day with soap for dark marks

Analysis:

- If you picked mostly *a*s, your skin is oily. The most obvious sign of oily skin is a shiny or greasy appearance all over the face. The oil may not appear immediately after washing but up to one to three hours later. You may need to wash your face several times a day to remove the excess oil. This excess oil will contribute to blackheads and frequent blemishes. Your pores will be very visible. You may see large yellow bumps on your skin that do not go away. These bumps are actually enlarged oil glands, called sebaceous hyperplasia.

- If you picked mostly *b*s, you have combination skin. You have oiliness across the forehead—often even when you pull your hair back—and down the nose and chin, but your cheeks remain normal or dry. You'll develop blemishes particularly in the T-zone area, and perhaps flakiness on the cheeks.

- If you picked mostly *c*s, your skin is most likely normal. This skin type will have some oil distributed throughout but no shine. After washing with a mild cleanser, your skin appears neither ashen or shiny. You typically don't need to wash or apply moisturizer to the face during the day, or you may use a light moisturizer only in the morning after cleansing. Blemishes may occur, but blackheads and prominent pores are infrequent.

- If you picked mostly *d*s, you have dry skin. It will feel tight after washing with even mild soap, and continue to feel tight throughout the day. Skin flaking, or ashiness, is also typical of dry skin. Your pores may be small and hard to notice. You will need to use a moisturizer on most days. Unfortunately, you may still develop acne.

- If you picked mostly *e*s, you have sensitive skin. This skin becomes easily irritated, itchy and red. You are prone to the development of a fine rash on the face.

You must select your facial and hair products carefully to avoid these reactions. In the past, you have probably applied over-the-counter hydrocortisone cream to the skin to remove the irritation.

• If you picked mostly *f*s, you have hyperpigmenting skin or skin with a marked propensity to develop hyperpigmentation. You must avoid products that can irritate the skin, produce rashes, or worsen acne. In addition to the hyperpigmenting characteristic, your skin may be dry, oily, or a combination of the two.

The main reason to determine skin type is to help you select the best products for your skin, including toners, moisturizers, and foundations. The skin-care programs described in chapter 2 will explain exactly how you can develop a regimen for your unique skin type in every season.

Skin-Type Variations in Women of Color

You may suspect that your skin has the characteristics of more than one skin type. Many women, for example, have oily facial skin but dry skin on the torso and extremities (lower legs, hands, and feet). That is simply because many of us have more oil glands on the face than on other parts of the body. As a woman, your skin type may also be affected by hormonal changes during the month or during different stages of life such as perimenopause and menopause (see chapter 13). If you travel frequently, your skin type may differ depending on the climate and sea level. Products and medications can also affect your skin type.

Skin of color, however, is more susceptible to seasonal changes. In fact, a survey conducted at the Skin of Color Center at St. Luke's Hospital in New York three years ago indicated that the majority of Black and Hispanic women studied had marked seasonal variations in skin type. In the winter, the skin of these women is often dry, tight, and ashen; in summer, the skin can be very oily and shiny. Similarly, the facial skin of these women who live in dry climates tends to be very dry while the skin of women who live in humid environments is oily. Depending on the season, the extremes of dry or oily skin types tend to predominate. You'll need to keep this in mind as you develop a skin-care and makeup routine.

A Closer Look at Sensitive Skin

Sensitive skin is simply skin that reacts easily to very common irritants, such as fragrances, dyes, oils, lanolin, soap, alcohol, chemicals, and preservatives. Sensitivity can affect any skin type. The signs include redness, itching, burning, or bumpiness that develop after product use. (Contrary to popular belief, foods rarely cause skin sensitivity.) Many women of color have skin that becomes easily irritated and dry in reaction to various common over-the-counter products. For Brown women, having sensitive skin can be especially troubling because the irritation may lead to pigmentation problems or the development of dark or light marks.

The good news is that some women who think they have sensitive skin actually don't. Your sensitivity may actually be explained by other skin conditions, such as eczema or seborrheic dermatitis, which can be treated. If you suspect you have sensitive skin or if you're not sure, consult a dermatologist. If in fact you do have sensitive skin, you'll have to be especially careful about what products you use on your skin and how you treat it. Here's what to avoid or use on sensitive skin only under a doctor's direction:

Toners or astringents containing alcohol
Products containing essential oils (concentrated oil extracts from plants)
Witch hazel
Moisturizers containing fragrance, lanolin, dye, vitamin E
Sunscreens containing fragrance, oil, PABA
Makeup containing oil
Alphahydroxy acid or retinol products (Retin-A)
Acne medications

Bleaching creams

Detergents and fabric softeners containing fragrance or preservatives

To protect your sensitive skin, shop for products and makeup with labels that say "alcohol-free," "fragrance-free," "hypoallergenic," "sensitive skin," or "non-comedogenic." A more detailed program for sensitive skin is described in chapter 2.

THE COLOR OF OUR SKIN

Anthropologists believe racial variations developed through natural selection, enabling early humans to adapt to particular environments. Darkly pigmented skin most likely developed to protect people living close to the Equator from ultraviolet (UV) light. (People living north of the Equator have paler skin to ensure absorption of UV rays that promote vitamin D formation in the skin.) An advantage that shielded our ancestors ages ago still guards us now from sun damage, skin cancer, and aging.

THE SUN AND OUR SKIN: WHAT YOU MUST KNOW

Many people of color believe the myth that because of our protective melanin, we don't get skin cancer. While it is true that we are far less likely to develop skin cancer than Whites—particularly the nonmelanoma forms of skin cancer—people of color do get skin cancer and when we do, we are more likely to die from this serious disease. In one paper on skin cancer that we wrote at the Skin of Color Center, we also showed that Black and Hispanic women who develop skin cancer had a higher rate of advanced disease than did Black and Hispanic men; it's not understood why.

For people of color, skin cancer can be a particular challenge for a number of reasons. The appearance and the location of skin cancer in a woman of color may be very different from the cancers (melanomas) that often affect Whites. Studies

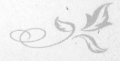

have found that melanomas in Blacks most often develop on the extremities—our palms, fingers, soles, toes—areas where a cancerous lesion may be easy to overlook. A common example of how melanoma may appear in skin of color is as a singular dark nail streak on the hands or feet.

　　To protect yourself, you must first be aware that you are at risk for skin cancer. Another way to protect yourself is to detect skin cancer early. Once every month, examine your skin from head to toe (see "Skin Self-Exam," below), paying particular attention to your hands, fingers, feet, toes, nails, and mouth, where melanoma-type skin cancers are more likely to appear in people of color. Look for dark brown or black spots in these areas, no matter how small. Pay particular attention to new spots or spots that change. The change can be an increase in size, shape, or color or a raised bump that develops within the spot. A bump on the foot or toe that is sore or does not heal is another tip-off for skin cancer. Be on the lookout for inklike spots or dark streaks along one nail only. Additional risk factors include age and a family history of skin cancer. (See the Skin Phototypes Chart that follows to assess your risk.) Finally, wear sunscreen with an SPF of at least 15 every day—not just when you go to the beach or on vacation. The sun exposure you receive simply from running daily errands may increase your risk of skin cancer.

Skin Self-Exam

The National Cancer Institute recommends these steps for checking your skin for signs of cancer. After a bath or shower, use a full-length or handheld mirror to check all areas, including your hands, feet, nails, mouth, and genitals. By checking your skin regularly, you will become familiar with what is normal. If you find anything unusual, see your doctor right away. The sooner skin cancer is found, the better chances for cure.

1. Look at the front and back of your body in the mirror, then raise your arms and look at the left and right sides.

2. Bend your elbows and look carefully at your palms, your fingers, your forearms including the undersides, and your upper arms.

3. Examine the back and front of your legs. Also look between the buttocks and around the genital area.

4. Sit and closely examine your feet, including the soles and the spaces between the toes.

5. Look at your face, neck, and scalp. You may want to use a comb to move hair so that you can see better.

SKIN PHOTOTYPES CHART

SKIN PHOTO-TYPE	UNEXPOSED SKIN COLOR	SENSITIVITY TO UVR*	SUNBURN/TANNING HISTORY	PHOTO AGING	SUSCEPTIBILITY TO SKIN CANCER
I	Ivory white	Very sensitive	Burns easily, never tans. Red hair, green eyes, freckles.	Strong; early onset	High risk
II	White	Very sensitive	Burns easily, tans minimally. Blond hair, blue eyes.	Strong; early onset	High risk
III	White	Sensitive	Burns moderately; tans gradually and uniformly. Brown hair, blue/hazel eyes.	Moderate to strong	Moderate risk
IV	Light brown	Moderately sensitive	Burns minimally; always tans well. Brown hair, brown eyes, olive complexion. Most light-skinned	Moderate to low; not excessive	Low risk

SKIN PHOTO-TYPE	UNEXPOSED SKIN COLOR	SENSITIVITY TO UVR*	SUNBURN/TANNING HISTORY	PHOTO AGING	SUSCEPTIBILITY TO SKIN CANCER
			Blacks, Asians, Latinos, and Native Americans.		
V	Brown	Minimally sensitive	Rarely burns; tans profusely. Most medium-skinned Blacks, Latinos, and Asians.	Slow, gradual, and low	Minimal or low risk
VI	Dark brown or Black	Least sensitive; insensitive	Never burns; tans profusely; deeply. Most dark-skinned Blacks.	Slow, gradual, and minimal	No risk

*UVR is ultraviolet radiation.

This chart is adapted from Fitzpatrick's Dermatology in General Medicine, *vol. 1; New York: McGraw-Hill, 1999, and* Beautiful Skin *by David E. Bank, M.D., et al., Avon, Mass.: Adams Media, 2000.*

Moles: What to Look For

We all have moles on our skin. Moles are simply growths or areas of skin where melanin-producing cells (melanocytes) are grouped together. To make sure your mole is just a mole, take note of the moles on your body—particularly new ones and ones that have changed—and ask the following questions:

Does it look like any other moles on my body?

Does it act like other moles on my body? (e.g., grow hair, etc.)

Has the mole recently changed in size, color, width, or texture?

Does the mole itch, tingle, bleed, or cause pain?

If you're concerned about a mole, be on the safe side. See a dermatologist for diagnosis and prompt treatment.

Office Visit: Do You Need to See a Dermatologist?

If you have a skin-care concern that over-the-counter products or a visit to your general practitioner or family physician does not resolve, make an appointment to see a dermatologist. You should definitely seek the care of a dermatologist if you have conditions such as acne, eczema, keloids, and hyperpigmentation (darkening of skin in patches or blotches), among others, to make sure you have the correct diagnosis and most up-to-date treatment. Get a referral from your physician or from friends. It's wise to choose a dermatologist who is either a person of color or who has had experience treating skin of color. To help your dermatologist zero in on the cause of your problem—and recommend an effective solution—I suggest you do the following:

- Jot down a description of the problem (use the form on page 29), including where the problem is located, how long you've had it, and how often it occurs. Be specific; instead of saying "I've had this symptom for a while," say "I've had it for three weeks . . ." List two things that make the problem better and two that make it worse. List any symptoms such as pain, itching, or bleeding.
- List the names and dosages of all medications you have recently used or bring all of the medicine to the visit in a plastic bag. Don't leave anything out—even birth control pills and vitamins can affect your skin.
- List and tell the doctor about any serious medical problems that you have or have had, such as cancer, diabetes, hypertension, or thyroid or kidney problems. List and tell the doctor if your are pregnant, nursing, or have recently delivered a baby.
- Bring along, in a plastic bag, all of the skin-care products you currently use, including cleansers, lotions, and makeup.

- Be sure to mention if there is a family history of the problem. Some skin conditions, such as lupus, eczema, and keloids, run in families.
- If you have multiple skin concerns, do not plan on discussing all of them during your first visit to the dermatologist—the physician may not have enough time to discuss all of them with you in one visit. Instead, begin with the problem that is bothering you the most.

Take This to Your Dermatologist

Description of problem and duration:

_____

_____

_____

_____

_____

_____

Medications and dosages:

_____

_____

_____

_____

_____

Family history of skin conditions/disease:

_____

_____

_____

_____

_____

Current skin conditions:

_____

_____

_____

_____

_____

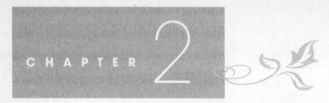

CHAPTER 2

GET WITH A PROGRAM: YOUR DAILY SKIN-CARE REGIMEN

To look your best every day, you need a daily skin-care regimen based not only on your skin type but also on the nature of your skin tone and the amount of melanin in your skin. Skin of color is very susceptible to developing either dark or light patches in response to a variety of factors. Everyday triggers such as sunlight, scratches, pimples, or even rashes can prompt the overproduction or underproduction of melanin, causing dark or light discolorations. To avoid the discolorations, you must treat your skin with great care. The way you tend to your skin every day can make the difference between a clear, glowing complexion and one with blotches or blemishes that can be difficult to camouflage or fade.

In this chapter, you'll learn how to put together a skin-care program, including ways to properly cleanse, exfoliate, tone, moisturize, and protect your skin. To make this program easy for you to adopt, I've summarized the steps in checklists, modified for skin type, at the end of the chapter.

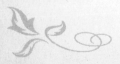

Cleansing Clues

- Cleanse your face daily to remove dirt, oil, and makeup.
- Avoid abrasive cleansers or cleansing products (puffs, loofahs), which can irritate skin of color.
- Use products designed for your skin type: oily, dry, normal, combination, or hyperpigmenting.
- Don't overdo it. Cleansing too often or too roughly will harm your skin.
- Exfoliate if you need to remove dull, dead skin cells by using exfoliating acids found in skin products—but test the product on a small patch of skin first.

COMING CLEAN: THE FACIAL STORY

To remove dirt, excess oil, perspiration, and makeup, most women of color should cleanse the face twice a day. The tools you select for washing are important. Think gentle. First, choose a mild, nonirritating cleanser. Avoid cleansers that contain abrasive granules for exfoliation. These harsh particles don't clean out pores and they can aggravate and irritate the skin, causing redness, or worse, darkening of the skin or hyperpigmentation. If you have acne, scrubbing with the granules can actually dramatically worsen an acne outbreak. Also, steer clear of acne puffs, loofah sponges, or rough washcloths. They will only irritate the skin.

Many women of color make the mistake of overcleaning—cleaning the face too often or too roughly. But most skin problems (acne, dark marks, clogged pores) are not caused by dirt, so there's no need to use harsh products or rough cleansing techniques. Also, our pigmented skin requires gentle care to avoid skin irritation that can trigger problems such as discoloration or even keloid scarring. Gentle cleansing with your fingertips or a soft cotton washcloth will do.

Beyond this general advice directed to all women of color, I suggest the following additional tips for women with different skin types. Remember, for many women of color, skin type tends to vary with the change of seasons. It's likely that most of you will change your cleansing ritual several times a year. Many will utilize the advice for oily skin in the hot and humid summer months of July and August and the advice for dry skin in the dry winter months of December and January. So remember, you may need to adjust your cleansing ritual and the products you use accordingly.

For Oily Skin. Wash your face two or three times a day to reduce excess oil. Avoid washing more than three times a day because this practice may irritate the skin, promoting low-grade inflammation of the skin and the subsequent development of dark patches. Wash early in the morning, immediately after work or school, and again just before bed. When washing, gently massage the face with a warm cleansing solution for one and a half to two minutes to dislodge the excess oil and skin debris. Use an antibacterial soap or a gel or foaming cleanser designed for oily skin (Cetaphil anti-bacterial soap, Avon Pore-fection cleanser, MD Forte Glycare Cleansing Gel) during the late spring, summer, and early fall months to remove excess oiliness, and a milder glycerin-based or oil-balancing soap or cleanser (Cetaphil for oily skin, Neutrogena Facial Cleansing Bar, Purpose soap, Basis All Clear Bar, pHisoderm Skin Cleansing Bar) in the winter and early spring months. Also, since oil on the forehead and temples can come from your hair, make some adjustment in your hair-care regimen. Try washing your hair at least once a week and wear it pulled or brushed back from the face. Avoid applying hair oils or pomades on the scalp near the forehead. They'll seep into the skin and produce more oil and shine.

For Combination Skin. Begin by washing the oilier areas of the forehead, nose, and chin first for one minute and then concluding with the dryer cheek area for a total cleansing time of one and a half minutes. This allows more time to be spent removing the oil and debris that has accumulated on the forehead, nose, and chin. As with oily skin, cleanse gently. Avoid washing more than twice a day. Consider using a light creamy cleanser, a nonsoap bar, or a glycerin soap, which attracts some moisture to the skin, twice a day during cooler seasons. One to try is Cetaphil Daily Facial Cleanser for Normal to Oily Skin or Purpose soap. Err on the side of a more emolliating (moisturizing) cleanser during the months surrounding winter because the cheek area and even the chin can become moderately dry at this time while the forehead and nose may remain slightly oily. In spring and summer, switch to a less emolliating cleanser such as the original Neutrogena glycerin bar on the cheeks as well as on the other facial areas because they will be oilier. Also, since oil on the forehead and nose can come from your hair, make the same adjustment in your hair-care regimen as outlined for oily skin. That is, try washing your hair at least once a week and wear it pulled or brushed back from the face. Avoid applying hair oils or pomades on the scalp near the forehead.

For Normal Skin. Because your skin is neither dry nor oily, you have flexibility in the products you choose, from Neutrogena for normal skin to Olay Cleansing Cloths. Wash your face twice a day if needed. However, if your skin becomes slightly oily or dry owing to weather change, follow the prescriptions for those skin types.

For Dry Skin. Despite what your mother may have taught you, wash your face only once a day unless you exercise or wear foundation or other makeup. If that is the case, it's important to wash the face at the end of the day to remove the pore-clogging makeup. Wash the facial skin gently with lukewarm water for about half a minute only. Use creamy cleansers that are emolliating to moisturize as you cleanse (L'Oreal Hydrafresh Cleanser, Cetaphil Gentle Skin Cleanser, Aveeno Moisturizing Bar for Dry Skin, Eucerin Gentle Hydrating Cleanser, Neutrogena Extra Gentle Cleanser). Switch to the richer, creamy cleanser products in winter and lighter versions in spring and summer. During the colder winter months, gravitate to products that do not produce a foamy lather such as Cetaphil or Aquinel—they will cleanse the skin without drying it out. Finally, for extremely dry facial skin, consider applying a cleansing product such as Cetaphil or Aquinel directly on the face and then removing the excess with a damp cotton pad, thus avoiding applying water directly to the face. The face will then have a satiny feel.

For Sensitive Skin. Wash once or twice a day with cleansers that are free of alcohol, lanolin, and fragrance (check the label). Also avoid cleansers containing benzoyl peroxide, salicylic acid, or glycolic acid. Avoid soap altogether if it irritates your skin. Cleansers to try are Olay Daily Facial Cleansing Cloths–Sensitive Skin, Dove Daily Hydrating Cleansing Cloths for Sensitive Skin, Sensitive Skin Dove, Olay Sensitive Skin, Neutrogena Extra Gentle Cleanser, and Cetaphil Gentle Skin Cleanser. While washing hair in the shower, tilt your head back to avoid getting potentially irritating shampoo or conditioner on your face. Don't forget to wash your hands frequently throughout the day and try not to touch your face. Your hands will transmit to your face the residue of all types of irritating products.

For Hyperpigmenting Skin. For skin of color that, with the slightest provocation, develops or forms dark marks, extra care must be given to the actual cleansing process and the selection of cleansing products. This skin should be cleansed no more than twice daily. Avoid washing with very cold or very hot water; use lukewarm or tepid water instead. Don't scrub or vigorously rub your skin. Products that produce tingling, stinging, or burning or that make the facial skin feel hot are to be avoided. Also skip products that cause the skin to turn pink or red after washing or that lead to visible peeling of the skin. Rely on cleansers designed for sensitive skin such as glycerin soaps like Neutrogena for Sensitive Skin, Olay for Sensitive Skin, or Dove for Sensitive Skin. Avoid products that contain irritants such as alcohol or benzoyl peroxide and salicylic acid.

Clean Up

Once you have your cleansing tools, take these steps to wash your face gently:

1. Create a lather or creamy mixture with your cleanser and lukewarm water.
2. Using your fingertips or a soft cotton cloth, gently massage the entire surface of your face for thirty to ninety seconds depending upon your skin type.
3. Rinse by splashing your face with water several times to completely remove dirt and cleanser residue—try to avoid extremely hot or cold water.

4. Carefully pat your face dry with a soft cotton towel—don't rub or pull on your skin to get it dry.

5. If you wear an oil-based or pressed-pancake type makeup, remove the makeup with a makeup dissolving cream (cold cream) before washing. Apply the cream and allow it to diffuse into the makeup for sixty seconds. Then with a soft cotton ball, applying minimal pressure, gently remove the makeup from the forehead. Do not rub the skin. Repeat this process with a clean cotton ball for each cheek, the nose, and chin. Finally, wash the face as indicated for your facial type (above).

Exfoliate

Your skin exfoliates, or sheds dead skin cells from the surface layer, naturally each day and even while you're sleeping. But the process of exfoliation may not be complete because skin cells sometimes stick together and remain on the face, leaving a dull, dry, and sometimes ashen appearance. Exfoliation may be accomplished at home either manually (with rough sponges, puffs, or gritty, granule-containing products on the body only) or chemically (with cleansers, creams, lotions, or gels containing exfoliating acids). If your complexion appears dull, you will benefit from regular exfoliation. To enhance exfoliation and cleansing, I recommend using products containing alphahydroxy acids (AHAs), polyhydroxy acid (PHAs), or betahydroxy acids (BHAs). An example of a widely used AHA is glycolic acid; the PHAs include nonglycolic fruit acids; salicylic acid is a BHA. These exfoliants come in cleansers, gels, lotions, creams, masks, and other skin-care products and are offered in a wide range of concentrations to suit individual needs. As long as exfoliants do not irritate the skin or trigger an allergic reaction, they can be used regularly.

As always, Brown women need to be especially careful when choosing these products. It's extremely important in skin of color to test a small area of your skin with the exfoliating product before using on a larger area or skin (see "Before You

Use That Product . . . ," below). Additionally, if you use any of these products, it's very important to let your doctor, aesthetician, or facialist know before any other products or medications are used on your skin.

Finally, harsh exfoliants that contain rough granules should be avoided in skin of color; they can irritate the skin and trigger pigmentation problems. That's why it's best to use exfoliants found in mild cleansers or other products if tolerated. If you are unable to tolerate the chemical exfoliants, then you can try the manual exfoliators. Ones to try may include Kiss My Face Organic Jojoba Mint Facial Scrub, Murad Purifying Face Scrub, or Nivea Visage Oil Control Cleansing Gel. If your skin becomes irritated after using any exfoliant, however, discontinue use and consult a dermatologist.

Before You Use That Product . . .

For women of color, it's especially important to perform patch tests on the skin before applying any potentially irritating products such as those containing exfoliating acids (alphahydroxy acid, etc.). To do a test:

1. Apply a small amount of the product to a small area of skin such as behind the ear, under the chin, or on the arm.
2. Leave the product on for twenty-four hours without getting the area wet.
3. Check the area for signs of irritation—redness, rash, burning, bumps, etc., after twenty-four hours and up to seven days. If you see any of these signs, do not use the product. Often you can return it to the store or manufacturer for a full refund.

Case in Point: Tender Loving Clean

Morgan, a sixteen-year-old with mild acne, came to see me with two complaints. First, she had bumps on her face, and second, her face hurt. On examination, I could see that her skin was red and irritated and that her acne was getting worse. When I asked about her skin-care routine, Morgan explained that she scrubbed her face three times a day (morning, afternoon, and at bedtime) with a maximum-strength acne wash. She also used either a rough washcloth or buffing sponge to get her face super-clean.

This harsh regimen was harming her skin. I instructed Morgan to wash her face only twice a day, using her fingertips, a mild nonmedicated cleanser (Cetaphil), and lukewarm water. She also began to moisturize with Cetaphil Lotion. I told Morgan that, in my opinion, buffing sponges were only good for scrubbing pots and pans! When she returned to my office a month later, she reported that her face was no longer red, irritated, or sore. And as I had anticipated, her acne had diminished as well, even without starting acne medication.

Do Extra Upkeep

For deeper cleaning, and a little self-pampering, you can add facials, steaming, or masks to your routine on a weekly or monthly basis, or for special occasions when you want your skin to look especially vibrant and clear. Local spas and beauty salons also offer these services performed by trained estheticians.

Steam Cleaning. Whether you do it at home or as part of a spa appointment, steaming your face with water vapor temporarily adds moisture to the skin's surface. This hydrating technique will not "open" your pores per se, but it will loosen dirt and dead skin cells, and give your skin a softer feel and a healthy glow. At home, you can simply place a towel over your head and lean over a bowl of just-boiled water flavored with two to three chamomile tea bags for five to ten minutes. At a spa, a technician may use a special machine to aim jets of steam onto your face. Whatever steaming technique you select, you must exercise caution so that the skin does not become burned. So do not place your face too close to the bowl, water, or jets of steam.

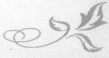

Behind Masks. Another way to exfoliate is by using a mild facial mask. Masks are not a necessary part of everyone's skin-care program, but if you like the way a mask leaves your skin looking and feeling, by all means use it. Look for a product formulated for your skin type. If you have oily skin, opt for a clay (kaolin) or mud mask that absorbs oil. Dry skin will benefit from a creamy, moisturizing mask. Avoid any products containing abrasives or granules that can irritate skin of color. Follow the instructions for the product and don't use more than once a week. Some products I recommend include M.D. Forte Skin Rejuvenation Hydra-Masque and Biore Blue Mask. If you prefer professional pampering, you can always schedule an appointment for a facial that includes a mask.

Facial Facts. In addition to relaxation, facials can help exfoliate the skin, clean pores, remove blackheads, and revitalize a dry or dull complexion. At a spa or salon, you have a number of options, including alphahydroxy acid facials and deep-cleansing facials. Ask your esthetician what facial type is best for your skin. Your treatment will start with a prefacial skin assessment under a magnifying lamp. In addition to the application of a cleanser, the facial treatment will probably include steaming, a light facial massage, manual removal of blackheads, and a facial mask. But be careful and ask questions before you undergo a full facial. For women of color the manual removal of blackheads (especially if they are deeply embedded) by the esthetician or facialist has the potential to produce discolorations or scarring. The technician should not push vigorously, pull, or pick the skin. If the blackhead does not pop out after the application of minimal pressure, then stop the procedure. Your dermatologist can prescribe medications that can remove the blackheads.

Selecting a Salon or Spa Professional

Beauty salons and spas abound these days, offering a great number of skin treatments. But because we have reactive skin, women of color

should choose salons or spas carefully. The esthetician, cosmetologist, or facialist who performs skin-care services should be licensed by your state board of cosmetology (go to http://www.beautytech.com/st_boards.htm to find the board in your state) and well trained. Be sure to ask whether she has knowledge and experience handling skin of color. Also find out whether the facility is supervised by a dermatologist certified by the American Board of Dermatology. Get referrals from friends and shop around before you settle on your salon.

To Tone or Not to Tone?

The purpose of skin toners is to remove surface oil, or sebum, from the skin. If you have very oily skin, a toning product can help clear your face of the grease that can clog pores and make them look larger. It can also minimize shine. How do you know whether or not you need to include a toner in your daily routine? If your skin tends to remain oily even after washing, or if your T-zone (forehead and nose) gets very oily, particularly in summer months, you may want to experiment with a toning product to see if it removes oil without irritation. After the application of a toner, your skin should not feel dry and tight. To the contrary, it should feel smooth, soft, and invigorated.

Many toners and astringents contain strong ingredients such as alcohol, which can aggravate sensitive, hyperpigmenting, or acne-prone skin, so choose the product carefully. (Witch hazel, though milder than alcohol, should also be avoided.) To get rid of the excessive oil safely, look for alcohol-free toners or astringents (Fashion Fair for Dry or Sensitive Skin, Neutrogena Clear Pore Oil Absorbing Astringent). The goal is not to use a toner that leaves your face taut, but one that will remove excess oil and leave the skin feeling smooth and silky. Once you've found the right toner, apply with a clean cotton ball, stroking the face gently to get a clean and completely dried face. Women with dry or normal skin do not typically need toners or astringents.

IT'S WISE TO MOISTURIZE

Moisturizers—creams, lotions, oils—work by attracting and trapping moisture and oil in the skin, leaving it soft and supple. They remove the dull, ashen appearance of dry skin that many women of color are prone to. A good moisturizer will also serve as a barrier between your skin and the elements, such as harsh wind and pollution.

Choosing the right moisturizer is key to keeping skin smooth while not clogging pores. Moisturizers come in a variety of types, including ones that are oil-based, water-based, oil-free, and vitamin-enriched. To choose the best moisturizer for you, you'll need to consider your skin type and seasonal change.

For Oily Skin. Women with oily skin can typically forgo a moisturizer. Yes, despite what your mother may have taught you, moisturizers will not prevent wrinkles (see "Sunscreen: The Skin Saver," page 46) and you will normally not need moisturizer unless your skin gets dry in the winter. In that case, opt for an oil-free formula that hydrates the skin. Consider products containing glycerin or other humectants that draw moisture to skin without clogging pores or imparting a greasy feel to the skin (Fashion Fair Oil Free Moisturizer).

For Combination Skin. Apply a light lotion once or twice a day to the dry areas of the skin only. You will probably not need to apply the moisturizer to the forehead and nose, which are typically oily. During the summer, switch to an oil-free product, such as Black Opal Oil Free Moisturizing Lotion, or eliminate it altogether.

For Normal Skin. You do not need to moisturize unless your skin becomes dry in winter or in certain climates. In that case, use an oil-free moisturizer like Black Opal Oil Free Moisturizing Lotion.

For Dry Skin. Moisturize two or three times a day, depending on your needs and your skin on a given day. During the fall and winter, use a rich cream or lotion designed for dry skin (Lancome Absolute Replenishing Crème SPF 15, Cetaphil Moisturizing Cream, Lubriderm Daily UV Lotion SPF 15, MD Forte Replenish Hydrating Cream—Hydra-Sorbet Aquatique, Moisturel Therapeutic Cream). Switch to a lighter lotion in the spring and summer. Avoid products containing vitamin A or retinol, which can further dry the skin. Also, steer clear of greasy products (Vaseline) that can clog pores, especially if your skin is acne-prone.

For Sensitive Skin. Follow the guide for oily, dry, or combination skin, but choose your moisturizer carefully. A water-based formula may be best. Avoid ingredients that can irritate your skin, such as alcohol, lanolin, retinol, vitamin A, PABA sunscreen, or fragrance. Products to try include Cetaphil Moisturizing Lotion, Keri Sensitive Skin, Lubriderm Seriously Sensitive Lotion, and Neutrogena Moisture for Sensitive Skin.

For Hyperpigmenting Skin. In general, moisturizing hyperpigmentation-prone skin—whether it's dry, combination, or sensitive—is important because excessive dryness of this type of skin can lead to itching, scratching, and discolorations. However, when selecting moisturizers it's best to avoid products with added ingredients such as vitamins, exfoliating acids (AHAs, BHAs), and benzoyl peroxide unless you patch-test your skin with these products. Those extra ingredients have the potential for inflaming the skin and then producing further hyperpigmentation. In other words, less is more. However, a moisturizer containing sunscreen, such as Olay Complete UV Protective Moisture Lotion or Aveeno Positively Radiant Daily Moisturizer SPF 15, may be beneficial in preventing sun-induced pigmentation. When selecting moisturizers for this type of skin, follow the guidelines for sensitive skin.

Extras

Many moisturizers on the market contain a host of additional ingredients you may or may not need. These include the following.

Vitamins. Vitamin-enriched products typically contain either vitamin C or E. These ingredients are considered antioxidants and may be beneficial for reducing sun damage and improving the appearance or the skin. Although preliminary studies may indicate improvement in the appearance of the skin with these products, many of the claimed benefits have not yet been proved definitively.

Vitamin A and retinol are often included in products for their anti-aging and anti-wrinkling properties. These products are beneficial in many cases, but excessive dryness and irritation of the skin can occur. Consult your dermatologist before selecting these products.

Additional supplements often included in skin-care products include coenzyme Q10, Kinerase, niacin, copper peptides, and alpha lipoic acid. These ingredients are touted for their possible anti-aging properties and may improve the skin's appearance in some women.

Alphahydroxy acids (AHAs). These acids exfoliate the top layer of skin. AHAs can reduce sun damage and acne and leave the skin with a wonderful glow, but overuse could irritate skin. I particularly like the MD Forte line of AHA products.

Sunscreen. Choosing a moisturizer containing sunscreen cuts out one step in your daily routine. The sunscreen should have an SPF of at least 15 in order to be effective.

Moisturizer Moves

To moisturize your facial skin effectively

- Apply the product directly onto damp skin after washing your face or showering. This way, the water is literally sealed into the top layers of your skin.
- Using your fingers, dot the moisturizer on forehead, cheeks, nose, and chin to ensure even distribution, then blend in.

DRY-SKIN TIP

Take shorter showers at lukewarm temperature. Then apply moisturizer directly onto damp skin.

BODY BEAUTIFUL

To keep your body skin soft and healthy, you need to give it attentive care. If you have dry skin—or any skin type during wintertime—practice the following routine: Bathe only once a day and limit showers and baths to five minutes. Use lukewarm water and minimize the amount of soap you apply. Olay Complete Moisturizing Body Wash contains petroleum and is good for very dry skin. Concentrate the lather under the arms and in the groin area. Don't forget to wash the soles of your feet, between the toes, and your ears. If you have sensitive skin, avoid cleansers with fragrances and skip the loofah or any other abrasive sponge. Keep a pumice stone handy and use on the feet daily or weekly depending on the condition of your feet. When you come out of the bath or shower, only pat your skin dry. Apply a moisturizer, such as Avon Moisture Therapy Body Lotion, Eucerin Plus Lotion, or Amlactin Lotion, to damp skin to trap moisture in the skin.

In summertime—or if you have oily to normal body skin—feel free to take lengthier showers or increase the temperature. You can also shower or bathe two

times a day. Loofah sponges are acceptable for exfoliation, but be careful not to make the skin raw or irritated.

If you are a plus-size woman, don't forget to lift your breasts and any abdominal folds and wash underneath. Also, lift each arm to wash armpits and one leg to cleanse the groin area. Pat your entire body dry with a towel and sprinkle the body folds with an absorbent powder like Zeasorb AF, which has antifungal properties.

If you have darkened areas on your neck and under the arms (*acanthosis nigricans*), dark elbows or knees, or small rough bumps on the arms and legs (*keratosis pilaris*), do not attempt to scrub the problem away. You'll only irritate the skin. (See below how to deal with dark elbows and knees.) If, however, you notice peeling skin on your towel, you may need to exfoliate manually (using a loofa) or chemically (using exfoliating acids). The following cleansers for the body offer a variety of options for women in color: Olay or Dove Bar Soap, Avon's Bath Gels, Olay Cleanser for Dry Skin, and Dove Cleanser.

Softening the Rough Spots

Regardless of skin type, you may have patches of dry skin in other areas, particularly your lips, elbows, knees, hands, and feet. Dry skin in these areas can become even more rough and ashy in winter months. To stay smooth all over, year-round, do the following.

Lips. Since the lips have few sebaceous or oil glands, they tend to become very dry, especially during the winter months. Licking the lips is not a solution since that practice will further dry the lips as the saliva evaporates into the air. Moisturizing the lips should become a regular part of your routine. Apply a lip balm or Vaseline to the lips several times a day. A lip balm that contains SPF 15 sunscreen is even better because it helps to prevent the lips from darkening in color from sun exposure—a problem for many Black women. A brand I recommend is Neutrogena Lip Moisturizer SPF 15, Avon Moisturizing Lip Treatment SPF 15 or Chapstick Lip Sensations. Applying moisturizing lipstick will also help keep your pucker soft all day. Finally, consider using an overnight lip-moisturizing product (Chapstick Overnight Lip Treatment) that you apply at bedtime and repairs cracked lips while you sleep.

Elbows and Knees. Exfoliate these areas daily by using a lotion or cream that contains glycolic acid, lactic acids, or urea. Examples include Eucerin Plus Lotion, Amlactin Lotion, or Carmol. If these areas are also darker in color than the surrounding skin on your arms and legs, as they often are in many Black women, apply a skin bleaching cream to lighten these spots after the lotion. (More on skin-bleaching products in chapter 3.) Don't rub or scrub the areas (they are not dirty) and try to avoid kneeling or leaning on the knees and elbows, which makes the problem worse.

Hands. Use only mild soap to wash hands as needed throughout the day and apply a rich lotion to moisturize. Because the cleansers in public washrooms are extremely drying, you should take a bar of mild soap in a soap dish to work with you to use in the ladies' room. Purchase a hand protectant such as Theraseal or Lipocream, and apply to hands throughout the day to provide a protective barrier between your hands and the environment. Wear rubber gloves when you wash dishes or perform wet housework. Remember to put thin white cotton gloves on (you can purchase them in any drugstore) before you put on the rubber gloves. The cotton gloves provide a barrier between your hands and the rubber gloves, which contain ingredients that can trigger an allergic reaction. Cotton gloves also absorb perspiration, preventing irritation and rashes. Try to avoid wearing latex or vinyl gloves for long periods of time and never wear them overnight. Carry a rich hand cream (Neutrogena Hand Cream or Avon Hand Cream) in your purse and apply it many times throughout the day, especially in cold weather. Be sure to wear cold-weather gloves throughout the winter to avoid dry, cracked hands. If you develop cracks in your fingers, apply a glob of Vaseline to the area several times a day. If they do not heal after a few days, then see your dermatologist for medicated ointments.

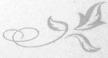

Feet. Use a pumice stone (usually found in the Dr. Scholl's section of the drug-store) in the shower every day to exfoliate the dry areas, typically the heels and balls of the feet. Rub the pumice stone on the surface of the foot very gently. Do not try to remove all of the dead skin in one session (this will only irritate your skin). Instead, remove a small amount each day for a month and then use it weekly for maintenance. Apply a rich moisturizer (Eucerin Lotion, Avon Intensive Dry Patch Stick, Amlactin Lotion, or Aquafor) while feet are still damp morning and night. If you have really rough, cracked heels and toes, soak your feet before bedtime in mild soap and lukewarm water, apply a thick moisturizer, and cover the feet with plastic wrap for two nights, then switch to cotton socks. They should be softer in a week. If the white flaky skin on the soles persists, you may have a fungal infection called *tinea pedis*. Consider applying an over-the-counter antifungal cream such as Lotrimin AF or Lamisil nightly for two weeks. If you see no improvement, consult a dermatologist. See a podiatrist for treatment of persistent corns or bunions.

Myth: Dry skin causes wrinkles.

Fact: Wrinkles are not caused by dryness, but by years of sun damage and facial expressions. To prevent wrinkles, apply sunscreen every day. Moisturizer can temporarily lessen the appearance of "fine lines."

SUNSCREEN: THE SKIN SAVER

Though the average woman of color has a natural SPF of 13 (which means we can stay in the sun without burning thirteen times longer than a White woman), we still need to include sunscreen in our daily skin-care program for four key reasons:

• Sun causes premature aging. Women of color are less susceptible to the signs of aging (wrinkles, sun spots), but we still age with at least some wrinkles, especially those of us with lighter skin tones.

- Sun causes sunburn. We are not immune to sunburns that damage the skin. Despite what many of us think, our skin can and will burn whether we go on a trip to the Caribbean, Mexico, or a local beach.
- Sun can contribute to skin discoloration. When stimulated by sun rays, our melanocyte cells can produce more melanin, triggering hyperpigmentation or darkening of the skin in uneven patches. If you already have dark marks on your face or body, the discoloration may become more pronounced.
- Sun suppresses the immune system. This effect probably weakens the body's ability to fight infection, cancer, and other conditions.

Sunscreens work by absorbing the harmful ultraviolet A (UVA) and ultraviolet B (UVB) rays before they can affect the skin. Sunblocks create a protective barrier that reflects UV rays, causing them to bounce off the skin. Like other skin-care products, sunscreens are formulated for different skin types. For most Brown women, a sunscreen with SPF 15 (which means you can stay in the sun fifteen times longer without burning) is sufficient, but if you have certain medical conditions, such as lupus, or take certain medications (see "Melanin and Medicine," page 14), you may need a sunscreen with SPF 30. Look for broad-spectrum products containing ingredients that protect the skin from both UVA and UVB rays. (Although women of color tend to avoid sunblocks that contain zinc oxide or titanium oxide because they leave a white coating on the skin, these agents provide the most complete protection from the sun.) Here's what more you need to know.

For Oily Skin. Choose a light sunscreen gel or spray such as Ombrelle Spray or Presun 30 gel. If you use moisturizer in cold-weather months, look for one that contains SPF 15 sunscreen.

For Normal/Combination Skin. Apply a sunscreen gel with SPF 15 or a sunscreen-containing moisturizer such as Aveeno Positively Radiant Moisturizer with SPF 15.

For Dry Skin. You can use just about any lotion or cream sunscreen—they stay on longer than gels. One I recommend is Cetaphil Daily Facial Moisturizer SPF 15. Your best bet may be a rich moisturizer containing sunscreen.

For Sensitive Skin. Shop for PABA-free, chemical-free sunscreens. (Sunscreens with zinc oxide or titanium oxide do make the skin look white, but newer products contain finer ingredients that fade into skin after several minutes.)

Sunscreen Steps

Be sure to apply your sunscreen after you've applied moisturizer or use a moisturizer that contains sunscreen. If you have an uneven skin tone, sunscreens are especially important. They will help protect your skin from further discoloration and speed the fading of dark marks. To maximize your protection, follow these guidelines:

- Always apply sunscreen twenty to thirty minutes *before* you're exposed to the sun to allow your skin to absorb the product and create a protective shield.
- Use sunscreen generously on all exposed skin—face, neck, and hands. Apply at least a shot-glass full (about one ounce) of the product.
- Store sunscreen away from the sun and heat to prevent spoiling.
- Reapply it after vigorous exercise or swimming even if the product is labeled "waterproof."
- Take note of expiration dates. If a bottle does not have an expiration date, toss it after one year.

Today, you can find sunscreen in a variety of skin-care products and makeup. However, one recent study demonstrated that sunscreen in foundation wears off after only a couple of hours. It's best to apply sunscreen separately, under makeup, or in moisturizers that say SPF 15 on the label.

Safe Beach Behavior

Tanning is never a safe activity. For Brown women, it often takes very little sun exposure to turn skin dark, and many experience a phenomenon known as "immediate tanning" or instant browning of the skin. But since many of us go to the beach with friends or family near home or while on vacation, we should be aware of the following sun-safe precautions:

- Apply SPF 30 sunscreen thirty minutes before going outside.
- Plan to spend all or most of your time at the beach before 11 A.M. or after 3 P.M., when the sun's rays are least intense.
- Wear light-colored clothing to reflect the sun's rays. Avoid wearing black clothing or black swimsuits, which absorb the sun's rays. Also consider washing your clothes in Sun Guard, a detergent that puts an SPF of 30 into the clothing.
- Wear a hat or visor and sunglasses to protect the eyes from UV rays.
- Stay under an umbrella in unusually hot weather.

First Aid for Sunburn

To soothe the pain of sunburn, take two aspirin every six hours and apply a cool compress, a cooling gel (containing aloe vera), or a topical anesthetic spray. A compress containing cold milk will reduce discomfort. An additional trick is to put the cooling gel in the refrigerator so that it will be cold on the skin.

DAILY SKIN-CARE PROGRAMS

Following the right skin-care program for your skin type will help you to properly cleanse, moisturize, tone, and protect your skin every day. Keep in mind that you may need to make adjustments as the seasons change. If, after following the program, you continue to have problems such as excessive oiliness, dryness, or frequent skin reactions (redness, breakouts), you may not have identified the right skin type. Or your skin type may have changed because of the weather. Refer to chapter 1 and review the information on skin types to make sure you've made the correct choice. Also, check whether the products you use regularly are actually suited to your skin type.

Oily Skin Program

- Cleanse your face two or three times daily with gel or foaming cleanser. You may select one containing glycerin, alphahydroxy acids, or betahydroxy acids. Pat skin dry.
- Apply an alcohol-free toner if oil persists after washing.
- Use an SPF 15 to 30 sunscreen spray or gel, or an oil-free moisturizer containing sunscreen.
- Wash hair at least once a week. Avoid applying hair oils or pomades near forehead. Wear hair back from face.
- Optional: Exfoliate weekly with a clay or mud mask made for oily skin.

Combination Skin Program

- Cleanse your face twice daily with a light, nonsoap bar or creamy cleanser. You may select one containing alphahydroxy or betahydroxy acids. Pat skin dry.
- Apply alcohol-free toner to the T-zone (forehead, nose, and chin) if oil persists after washing.
- Use an SPF 15 to 30 sunscreen gel, or a light oil-free lotion containing sunscreen, particularly on the cheeks.
- Wash hair weekly. Avoid applying hair oils or pomades near forehead. Wear hair back from face.

- Optional: Exfoliate weekly with a combination of masks—one made for oily skin on the T-zone and the other moisturizing mask on the cheeks.

Normal Skin Program

- Cleanse your face up to two times daily with a light cleanser made for normal skin.
- Apply an oil-free moisturizer only if needed in cold weather.
- Use an SPF 15 to 30 sunscreen gel, or a light oil-free lotion containing sunscreen.
- Optional: Exfoliate weekly with a mask made for normal skin.

Dry Skin Program

- Cleanse your face once daily with a creamy moisturizing cleanser. Wash again at night if you wear makeup.
- Moisturize, while skin is still damp, with a rich cream or lotion twice daily or more.
- If you have not already, apply an oil or cream sunscreen, SPF 15.
- Optional: Exfoliate weekly with a creamy, moisturizing mask.

Sensitive Skin

- Cleanse once or twice daily with an alcohol-free, lanolin-free cleanser.
- Apply a light, water-based moisturizer free of alcohol, lanolin, PABA sunscreen, or fragrance.
- Use a PABA-free, chemical-free sunscreen with SPF 15.
- Optional: Exfoliate weekly with a gel mask containing very mild ingredients, such as aloe.

Hyperpigmenting Skin

- Cleanse no more than twice daily with an alcohol-free, lanolin-free cleanser and lukewarm water.
- Apply a light, water-based moisturizer free of alcohol, lanolin, PABA sunscreen, or fragrance.
- Use a PABA-free, chemical-free sunscreen with SPF 15.

Minimalist's Routine

Many busy women of color don't have the time or the desire to spend several minutes in front of the mirror each morning with a time-consuming program. To keep your daily routine to a minimum, all you need are two essential products. Shop for a cleanser designed for your skin type and moisturizer with sunscreen (just sunscreen for oily skin). You can supplement this minimalist's regimen with weekly masks.

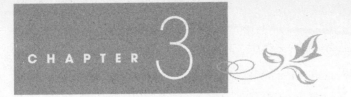

CHAPTER 3

COLOR ME BEAUTIFUL

From the days you first experimented with your mother's lipstick or painstakingly applied eye shadow or eyeliner, you've known the pleasure and fun of using cosmetics to enhance your looks. But as a woman of color you've probably also known the frustration of trying to find just the right shade of foundation, blush, or lipstick for your unique skin tones. Until recently, few cosmetics companies created makeup with our wide array of skin tones in mind. Even today, with a number of cosmetic brands formulated for women of color (Iman, Black Opal, Fashion Fair) and some mainstream companies offering a wider choice of colors (Revlon, Avon, Mac, Bobbi Brown, Prescriptives), it may still be difficult to find the appropriate shades of makeup to flatter our skin.

Do the cosmetics you currently use help you look your best? If you suspect you could benefit from making some adjustments or major changes, read on. You don't need to settle for a not-quite-right shade of foundation or a powder that is a little too light or too dark for your skin. And you don't necessarily need an elaborate, time-consuming routine or expensive brands. The more you learn about your skin and how to properly complement it with cosmetics, the easier it will be to select and use the most flattering products. Choosing all your makeup from one brand may not be the best strategy. But a little experimentation and willingness to

change what you've been doing all along might give a boost to your looks and to the way you feel about yourself.

In this chapter, I'll share with you what I know about choosing foundations and other products. You'll learn what makeup items every woman needs, how to put together your basic look, and how to camouflage certain imperfections, such as dark marks, with makeup. I'll answer some common questions women of color have about applying makeup. And if you don't like wearing much makeup and prefer a more natural look, this chapter will speak to you, too.

COSMETICS: THE CHALLENGE FOR WOMEN OF COLOR

Why is it often so difficult for women of color to find correct cosmetic shades and apply them creatively to look our best? There are a number of reasons. One is that most cosmetic companies offer a limited palette of foundation, blush, and lipstick colors for all women to choose from. Considering the estimated thirty-five different skin hues or shades among women of just African descent, it's no wonder that these companies do not often satisfy our needs! While some cosmetics companies have created makeup product lines for women of various ethnicities, giving us more options than ever, there's still a lack of "diversity" in cosmetic shades that truly reflects the variety of skin tones among us.

Another challenge for us is uneven skin tones. Because women of color tend to be more prone to pigmentation discolorations, we face the added challenge of having to diminish and camouflage dark or light patches in our skin. If the degree of discoloration is significant, simply applying multiple layers of foundation or powder will not achieve the effect we want. Because of tanning and sun damage, many of us also have variations in tone between the face, neck, and chest, making the selection and application of foundation color even trickier.

Adding to these difficulties is the fact that many women don't understand the

role of foundation and how to apply it. Foundation should be selected to give the facial skin a smoother, more even appearance and enhance—not cover up—your natural beauty. You'll want to select a shade that most closely approximates your natural skin tone—not one that is slightly lighter or darker—and apply it evenly, or your complexion will have an artificial or "made up" appearance. To select the correct color, you not only need to match the overall tone of your skin but also identify your skin's undertone. This information will help in choosing the best concealer, powder, blush, and other cosmetics for your skin tone and type.

A Quick Story

During my early twenties I used a Revlon foundation daily even though the shade was not the best match for my skin tone and was inappropriate for my oilier skin type. Why was I using this particular foundation? Because it was the brand and shade my mother used. Both the shade and degree of moisturization were perfect for my mother's skin. I didn't consider seeking a more appropriate foundation for my skin until I went to college. One day my roommate and I went to a department store and asked a clerk at the Fashion Fair cosmetics counter to apply their foundation to our skin. At that time, it was a much better match in terms of color and it was also less oily for my combination skin.

The lesson for me that day was to experiment in order to find the best products for *my* skin. Now I select from ten different types of foundations, including several brands: two each from Bobbi Brown, Avon, Black Opal, Fashion Fair, and Olay. One set is for summertime when my complexion is darker and the other for winter when I turn more pale. The different brands also contain varying amounts of oil. For example, when my skin feels dry, I apply the moisture-rich Bobbi Brown and when I feel oily, I choose Black Opal. You too should feel free to use different products from different brands to find the best mix of cosmetics for your skin.

Tones and Undertones

The tone of your skin is its predominant surface hue or shade. Brown women's skin tones generally fall into the broad categories of dark brown or black, brown, and light brown or beige, with many variations in between. The undertone is an underlying hue or color that is less visible (almost beneath the surface of the skin), but it is important because it modifies the overall tone, giving a richness to skin color. Women of color have a greater variety of undertones than White women. The undertones that tend to dominate among us are yellow, orange, and red, but some of us also have olive or blue undertones as well.

Understanding your undertone is a key step in selecting the most flattering makeup shades. If you apply a foundation that matches your skin color but not the undertone, it can make the makeup look unnatural, even garish. When it comes to foundations, the most common complaint I hear from women of color is that the foundation has undertones that are too orange or too red for their skin.

How do you identify the correct undertone of your skin? You may be able to tell simply by looking at the skin on your neck, which gives your true color because it's less affected by the sun's rays. Or consult a trained makeup consultant at your local cosmetics counter, who should be able to tell you what the undertone is and how to choose cosmetic shades accordingly. Many of these counter consultations are free of charge, but check first to find out what the service involves. And remember, it's important to experiment. You might also contact your local spa or salon to see if it offers makeup consultation and application. (See "Makeup Match-Up," page 70.)

Seasonal Shifts

It's important to remember that your skin tone is likely to be different during summer months than in winter, even if you don't purposely go to the beach to tan. Many women of color experience a phenomenon called "immediate tanning," which means their skin can sometimes turn dark very quickly with even just a few minutes in sunlight (walking down the street or driving in a car on a sunny day). Even a slight darkening of skin color during spring and summer will cause your skin tone to clash with the foundation you used during fall and winter, giving you a less than optimal look.

For that reason, like many women of color, you'll need more than one foundation—a color that matches your natural complexion (without any tan) and another that is one or more shades darker depending on the degree of tan you typically experience in warm weather. Consequently you'll also need to adjust your concealer and powder shades. (Considering the fact that you may only need to replace these products every six months to a year, the cost is not prohibitive.) For example, I use Bobbi Brown foundation #6 in the middle of summer when my skin is darkest and foundation #5 during the winter when I'm paler. I also switch between two different shades of Fashion Fair powder, which have enough yellow undertones to match my skin, unlike the Bobbi Brown #3 powder, which has an orange pigment that does not match my undertones. So don't be afraid to use products from different lines. Mixing and matching will allow you to find the perfect concealer, foundation, and powder for your skin.

MASTERING MAKEUP

To get a polished look, I suggest you use concealer, foundation, powder, lipstick, and perhaps mascara. For a more striking appearance, you may want to add eyeliner, eye shadow, lip liner, and blush. But the goal is not to look painted—it's to enhance your true beauty. How much makeup you use is a matter of personal preference. Here's what you need to know about choosing and using the right cosmetics. The product recommendations in this chapter include my own suggestions and those of women of color makeup artists I've consulted.

Concealer Clues. The purpose of concealer is to conceal or camouflage darker areas of the face (such as the under-eye area) and blemished or blotchy spots. The color of your concealer should be a shade lighter than your foundation—that is, a shade lighter than your natural skin tone. After cleansing, moisturizing (if needed), and applying sunscreen to your face, dot concealer in your trouble spots. Use a light touch—too much concealer can give your complexion an uneven, cakey look. You can use a damp makeup sponge or your fingers to blend in. Don't rush the blending process—take your time to get the right, even-toned look. Try a MAC concealer or Bobbi Brown or MAC full coverage foundation as concealer.

Foundation Facts. Foundation is used to even out skin tone and give your face a smooth appearance. Choosing the correct color is crucial, so be sure to test a product before you buy it. To do this, have the makeup consultant apply the foundation to your entire face, and take a good look at your skin in natural light. (The foundation will appear different under artificial light; see "Foundation Tip," page 60.) If the foundation blends in and disappears, thus appearing natural, it's the right color. A too-light foundation may make your skin look ashen. Take a closer look to make sure the foundation's undertone is not too red, orange, or yellow. If the color does not match, keep trying other shades, either from that line of cosmetics or from an altogether different line, until you find the one that most closely approximates your skin tone.

The next step is to make sure you've chosen a foundation for your skin type. This is important because the wrong type can make the skin look dull or too shiny—or worse, like you're wearing a mask. Foundations come in different forms—liquid, cream, cream-to-powder, and stick, matte and moisturizing formulas. If you have acne, you'll need a light oil-free foundation that doesn't clog your pores and trigger a breakout. Avoid oil-based products, such as those often found in compacts, and opt for nonacnegenic or noncomedogenic products instead. Whatever your skin type, you may need to switch products when the seasons change or if you move to a dry climate.

For oily skin. Look for oil-free or water-based foundations, or a foundation and powder in one compact. Matte or semi-matte formulas will look best on your skin. If you have very oily skin, don't forget to use a toner before applying any makeup and blot oily areas during the day with tissue. Try Estée Lauder's Double-Matte Foundation for oil control. Avon's Clear Finish Oil-Free Foundation, an antiacne treatment that contains salicylic acid, is perfect for acne-prone skin as well as oily skin.

For normal/combination skin. A water-based foundation should suit your needs. If you have T-zone skin and your cheeks become especially dry, experiment with water-and-oil combination products. Semi-matte formulas will look best.

For dry skin. Opt for moisturizing foundations that contain some amount of oil or a combination of oil and water—but only if you are not acne-prone. These often come in cream or liquid form. For acne-prone skin, oil-free foundation is still best. Just apply a moisturizer before applying your foundation.

For sensitive skin. As always, choose hypoallergenic products that are free of potential irritants. A light, water-based foundation should do.

For hyperpigmenting skin. Since this skin type is prone to the development of dark marks, camouflaging the marks with foundation is essential. Consider using a foundation stick, such as Black Opal Stick Foundation, or a foundation in a compact, such as MAC Studio Fix Powder Foundation, for more complete coverage.

How to Apply Makeup

Use a round or wedge-shaped cosmetic sponge, or your fingers, to dot about a nickel-size amount of foundation along the forehead, cheeks, nose, and chin, then blend in evenly.

Because of the difficulties in finding the right foundation color, some makeup experts believe that Brown women should use more than one foundation shade by blending two shades together or by applying different shades to different areas of the face (one shade on the T-zone area and another on forehead, cheeks, and jaw, for example). Some women prefer to have their foundations custom-blended. In my opinion, it's often too difficult for women to blend makeup on their own and get consistent color. Custom blending, like that offered by companies like Prescriptives, is a tremendous advance for Brown women because you can leave the store with one bottle that is made just for you. However, the downside is higher cost. If you have not been able to find a color that suits you on your own, consult a cosmetics counter or makeup artist for expert advice.

Foundation Tip

When selecting foundation, test the color on the skin of your entire face and not just along your jawline (which is difficult to see in the mirror). Don't test it on the back of your hand because this skin is a different color and texture from facial skin. Most important, view the shade under natural light: leave the store and go outside to decide if the shade is perfect for you.

Powder Perfect. Powder is an important step to enhancing your natural beauty. It enables you to enhance your foundation, get more complete coverage, give more polish to your look, and make makeup last longer. You can also use powder in a compact to touch up your complexion throughout the day. Powder is well worth the investment. Like foundation, powders come in different forms—loose, finely milled powder, or pressed, cakey powder. The key to your selection is, again, skin type.

For oily skin. Select a loose powder that is formulated to absorb oil. Pressed powders may clog pores. Try MAC blot powder to control oil.

For normal/combination skin. Use a loose or pressed powder. If you have T-zone skin, select a nonoily moisturizing product. Look to Fashion Fair pressed powders.

For dry skin. Your best bet is a moisturizing pressed or loose powder.

For sensitive skin. Buy a hypoallergenic loose powder for your skin type.

For hyperpigmenting skin. Select a powder for your skin type whether it is oily, dry, or normal skin. Opt for pigmented powder if your dark marks are not fully camouflaged by foundation.

Powders may be translucent (sheer) or pigmented to match the color of your foundation. For many women, translucent powder will suffice. You may want to use a pigmented powder if you have skin discolorations or unevenness that are still visible; make sure, however, that the powder hue truly blends in and is not too orange or red. MAC or Guerlain bronzing powders have a nice effect. Use a large makeup brush or powder puff to apply the powder evenly over your face.

Ideal Eyes. To accent your eyes, you can use eye shadow, eyeliner, and mascara as well as eyebrow makeup.

Wow brows. Well-defined, neat brows provide a natural frame for your eyes and face. Before applying any eye makeup, make sure your brows are groomed. If you have thick brows or excess hair between them, consider getting a professional wax or invest in a good tweezer, but be careful not to overpluck. Long-term overplucking may result in the hair never growing back, which can be a problem if you wish to change the shape of your brows or if you decide on a fuller look. If you have very thin brows, do not attempt to "draw" in a straight or arched brow line; this looks very artificial. Instead, after grooming your brows with an eyebrow comb, brush on light strokes of eyebrow pencil or eye shadow that match the color of your hair to add depth and color. A mix of pencil and shadow will give you a more natural look. Brands to try are Fashion Fair or Lancome brow pencils or MAC #263 angle brush with any of their medium to dark brown shadows.

Super shadows. Eye shadows can subtly accent the eyes or highlight them dramatically. You may use two to three different shades to achieve the effect you desire—an overall neutral shade similar to your skin tone, a slightly darker color on the lid, and a darker shade in the crease. Powder shadows are the easiest to use; apply with a shadow applicator that comes with the product or with a thin makeup brush. Then blend colors. Recommended brands are MAC, which offers a wide range of colors, Make-up Forever, and NARS.

Silver lining. You can literally draw more attention to your eyes by applying eyeliner to the lids, under the eyes, or in both places. You'll have the most control and a more natural look with a pencil liner. With a steady hand, draw or dot the liner from the outer edge of the eye inward. For a more dramatic look, try a liquid liner or eye shadow applied with a moistened makeup brush. The key to a neat, soft line is practice. Recommended brands are MAC Smoulder Eye Pencil, Bourjois liquid liner, Lancome Art Liner, and Avon liquid liner.

Mascara mystique. The final step in eye makeup application is the mascara. Before applying mascara, you may want to curl your lashes with a lash curler, but this may not be necessary for everyday makeup. Then sweep the mascara wand along the length of your lashes, allow to dry, and apply a second coat if necessary. If the mascara clumps, use an eyelash comb to separate lashes and remove excess makeup. Recommended brands include MAC Pro Lash and L'Oreal Voluminous Waterproof Mascara. If you want to try false eyelashes, be careful not to get the adhesive in your eye. Be aware that some women experience an allergic reaction to the adhesive, which is characterized by itching, swelling, and redness of the eyelids. If that occurs, stop using the eyelashes immediately.

RED EYE

Are your eyes sometimes red and itchy? The culprit may be an allergy to your eyeliner, mascara, or the adhesive that glues false eyelashes to your lids. Stop using the product for two weeks to see if symptoms subside. If an allergy is the problem, you may need to shop for hypoallergenic eye makeup or use a natural alternative. For example, a coat of Vaseline on your eyelashes is a great alternative to mascara.

SHELF LIFE

How long has your mascara been in your makeup bag? If you can't remember, you probably need to replace it. If you've used the same mascara for a year or longer, it's now a breeding ground for bacteria.

Blushing Beauty. Blush, also known as rouge, can be used to warm the face and emphasize your cheekbones. They come in different forms (powders, creams, gels, mousses) and a wide variety of colors. Your selection should be based on your style and the look you want to achieve. Don't be afraid to try colors outside of the range you're used to—you may be surprised to see how flattering neutral shades such as bronze look on our skin. Before selecting a blush, make sure it is made for your skin type. Use a medium-size makeup brush or sponge to blend powder blush from hairline to cheek and on temples. Apply the blush just below your cheekbone for maximum effect. Some recommended brands that offer a great range of colors include Ben Nye, Fashion Fair, and MAC.

A Pretty Pout. With lip liners, lipsticks, and gloss you have the tools to create a lovely mouth that can speak volumes.

Lining up. Why bother with lip liner? It can help accentuate your lips, reshape an uneven lip line, and keep lipstick from bleeding. Choose a liner that matches your lipstick color; outline the shape of your mouth with the pencil. You can change the shape of an imperfect pout by patting foundation around your lip lines and drawing a line inside or outside the natural line to create the illusion of evenness. Lip liner can also be used in place of lipstick for a more natural look.

Lipstick lowdown. Perhaps the easiest part of your makeup routine is applying the lipstick. Lipsticks come in an array of shades and three general formulations: matte (smooth, no shine), semi-matte (subtle shine), and cream or moisturizing (glossy shine). Matte shades tend to give a more dramatic, movie-star appearance to the face, but they can be drying to the lips. Semi-matte and moisturizing lipsticks give a softer appearance to lips. After lining the lips with liner (above), stroke lipstick over the entire mouth, including the liner, being careful not to go outside your lip lines. Blot with tissue and reapply. Brands to try for great color variety are Avon, MAC, and Sephora.

Lip gloss. Used alone or in combination with liner and lipstick, lip gloss adds shine and softness to the lips. Many women these days use gloss alone in nude or neutral shades (beige, cinnamon, mocha) for a low-maintenance look. Or you can apply a matte or semi-matte lipstick to the lips and dot gloss in the center for subtle shine. Recommended products include Kiels, Bourjois glosses, and MAC lip gloss or lip lacquers. Other top picks include Lancome Juicy Tubes, Cargo Lipgloss, and Aveda Brilliant Lip Shine.

Dry Lip Tip

If your lips are frequently dry, cracked, or peeling owing to cold weather or drying matte lipsticks, add a lip balm to your routine. Apply a lip balm or Vaseline before applying lip liner and lipstick to protect lips from the elements and wear-and-tear of makeup usage. In the summer, apply an SPF 15 lip balm. Also use an overnight lip treatment to repair your dry, cracked lips while you are asleep, such as Chapstick Nighttime. Another good choice is MAC lip conditioner. To gently remove the dead skin, use a child's soft toothbrush once or twice a week. Do not pull the dead skin off.

Two-tone Lips?

Many women of color have lips that are two completely distinct shades—a darker shade on top and a lighter, more pink or reddish shade on the bottom. But you don't need two shades of lipstick to get an even-toned look. Instead, try filling in the lips with liner before applying lipstick to help even out the different tones or apply a small amount of foundation to your lips before applying your lipstick.

ADDED VALUE

Many lipsticks these days contain more than color. To protect your pucker from the elements and keep lips soft, look for additional ingredients such as sunscreen and aloe.

COLD SORE ALERT

If you are developing or have developed a cold sore, do not use your lip products. You will contaminate the products and be unable to use them in the future.

Makeup Recap

To create a polished look for weekdays, follow these steps after you've washed your face and applied moisturizer (for dry or combination skin) or toner (oily skin) and sunscreen:

1. Apply concealer (one shade lighter than your natural skin tone) to blotchy or uneven areas using fingers or a makeup sponge to camouflage discolorations. Blend.
2. Apply foundation (the same color as your skin) by dotting it all over the face and blending evenly with a makeup sponge to create a smooth, even complexion.
3. Dust a layer of translucent powder (or pressed powder the same color as your foundation) over the face with a makeup brush or powder puff to set foundation.
4. Apply eye shadows, eyeliner, and/or mascara to accent your eyes.
5. Apply blush just below cheekbones with a makeup brush or sponge.
6. Apply lip liner and two coats of lipstick for the finishing touch.

The Minimalist's Makeup Routine

1. Apply concealer to uneven areas, like under the eyes, and blend.
2. Wipe a combination powder-foundation formula in a compact over the face.
3. Apply lipstick.

Case in Point: Makeup and Acne

Claire, a thirty-five-year-old woman of Caribbean descent, had been battling acne for years before she came to my office. She told me she experienced frequent outbreaks throughout each month but especially before her period. Claire complained not only of acne bumps but also of dark areas on her forehead, cheeks, and chin. To camouflage the dark spots, she'd apply several layers of a heavy, oil-based foundation each morning and even apply more layers throughout the day. I explained to her that her foundation was one cause of her frequent acne flare-ups because the oils in her foundation exacerbated the condition. Additionally, since her foundation was so thick, Claire would vigorously scrub her face each night to remove the makeup. By doing that, she was irritating her skin and inadvertently making her acne worse.

Claire agreed to let go of her cherished foundation. I recommended that she first apply a concealer to the dark areas, then an oil-free liquid foundation followed by a light dusting of powder to cover her blemishes and even out her complexion. At the same time, I prescribed the acne medications Benzaclin Gel and Differin Gel, and a hydroquinone bleaching cream, Lustra AF with sunscreen, to diminish the dark marks. As her acne improved, Claire developed fewer dark areas and those she had began to fade.

Your Makeup Tool Kit

What you need:

- Concealer

- Foundation (at least two, one for high-sun-exposure and one for low-sun-exposure seasons)
- Powder (loose or pressed and in a compact)
- Cosmetic sponges, wedge-shaped or round
- Makeup brushes of varying sizes for powder, blush, and eye shadow (recommended are Trish McEvoy brushes, MAC #263 or #224 brushes, or Bobbi Brown brush set)
- Eyebrow grooming comb
- Tweezers
- Makeup remover

Don't Leave Home Without It

To be prepared for any event, be sure to carry these must-have makeup savers:

- Tissues for blotting oiliness and lipstick
- Compact containing powder or powder-foundation
- Lipstick or lip gloss

Removing Makeup

Though makeup does fade during the course of the day, you still need to remove it thoroughly at night, especially if the makeup is oil-based. If you don't completely remove your makeup daily, it can attract dirt, clog pores, and cause breakouts. Women who use water-based products may be able to remove all of the makeup with the same cleanser used on the face in the morning. However, oil-based makeup used on dry or combination skin will need to be removed with a makeup removal product. One brand to try is Dermablend Remover/Nettoyant.

Makeup removers are formulated for skin type. Once you've selected one for your skin, apply the product according to instructions. You may need to leave it on your skin for several minutes to give it time to dissolve the cosmetics. Use tissue or cotton balls to *gently* wipe away the residue. Cotton swabs may be more useful for the sensitive eye area (but avoid cotton if you wear contact lenses). Take care not to tug or pull at your skin. If makeup does not come off, you may need to apply additional remover or switch to a more effective product. Women with sensitive skin should avoid products containing irritants such as alcohol and fragrance.

To make makeup removal easier and less time-consuming, you may want to avoid using "waterproof" products like mascara. "Water resistant" mascara does not last as long and may smudge more readily, but it is more easily removed than a waterproof product. (Also, how often do you go swimming with mascara on?) Pencil and powder eyeliner or eyebrow makeup will be easier to remove than liquid products. (If you wear contact lenses, look for eye makeup labeled "for contact-lens wearers" to avoid irritation.) Your choice of makeup formulas depends, of course, on personal preference, but consider the time you're willing to devote to makeup removal before you buy.

Makeup Storage and Care

How you store and maintain your makeup and makeup tools will make a difference in your looks. If you keep makeup too long it can affect the quality and color of the product as ingredients age and as oils from your fingers and face mix with the cosmetics. It can also allow bacteria or fungi to grow and cause infections, most commonly of the eye or lip. Your makeup tools—brushes, sponges, applicators— can also become filled with makeup and oils, interfering with clean makeup application and creating another breeding ground for bacteria. To keep your makeup fresh and clean, get in the habit of taking these steps:

1. Replace all eye makeup (liner, shadows, mascara) every three to six months. Liquid products should be tossed every three months.
2. Replace other makeup (foundation, powder, concealer, lipstick) every twelve months.

3. Wash makeup tools every two weeks in mild soap and warm water. Air-dry.

4. Replace makeup sponges once a month.

5. Stop using lipstick, lip liner, gloss, and balm if you develop a cold sore or fever blister. Replace the products if you accidentally use them during an infection.

6. Replace all eye makeup if you have had conjunctivitis or "pink eye."

7. Store all makeup products in a dry, cool environment. Keep products tightly closed.

CLEANUP TIP

If you can apply your powder, blush, or eye shadows without dipping into the makeup, it's time to clean your makeup brushes.

KEEP IT CLEAN

This chart will help guide you in the care of your makeup, skin, and eyes. When in doubt, use common sense. If a makeup product begins to clump, changes consistency or color, or emits an odor, play it safe and throw it out. Liquid and cream products should generally be replaced more frequently than powder products.

PRODUCT	HOW LONG TO KEEP
Foundation	1 year
liquid foundation	6 months–1 year (or if it separates)
Powder	1–2 years
Blush	1–2 years
liquid rouge	1 year
Eyeliner	3–6 months
liquid eyeliner	3 months
Mascara	3 months
Eye shadow	1 year
Lipstick	1 year (or if oil beads appear, or odor or color changes)
Makeup sponges	1 month (unless washable)

Makeup Safety Tip

Never use makeup testers in department stores. If even one person has touched the item, bacteria may be present.

Makeup and Allergies

Occasionally, makeup ingredients can trigger allergic reactions. These reactions most commonly occur on the upper and lower eyelids from eye makeup such as eyeliner and mascara because of the preservatives these products contain. Signs you may have a makeup allergy may also include a rash, swelling, or excessive wrinkling of the skin around the eyes. Also, you may develop a sudden breakout on the skin or a rash around the lips (owing to dye in some lipsticks). If you notice a reaction, stop using the product immediately. Take an antihistamine to relieve symptoms if the reaction persists. If reactions continue no matter what product you use, schedule an appointment with a dermatologist or an allergist. The physician can administer an allergy patch test to determine what specific ingredient your skin may be reacting to. One way to avoid potential triggers of allergic reaction is to patch-test the product on your skin before use. If you are allergic to your mascara, you might try applying a small amount of petroleum jelly (Vaseline) to lashes for a fuller, thicker appearance.

MAKEUP MATCH-UP

As a woman, I've learned to work with different makeup brands to match my skin tone, undertone, and type. As a dermatologist, I've talked to numerous makeup artists to find out more about which brands are most often recommended for matching the tones of women of color. Use this guide to start your search for the products that work for you.

SKIN TONE	UNDERTONE	CELEB EXAMPLES	MAKEUP ARTIST RECOMMENDED BRANDS
Light beige	Yellow		MAC, Bobbi Brown, Estée Lauder
Beige	Yellow gold	Veronica Webb	MAC, Bobbi Brown, Estée Lauder
Tan/olive	Medium yellow/green		MAC, Bobbi Brown, Fashion Fair
Light brown	Medium yellow/ orange/red	Halle Berry	Bobbi Brown, Fashion Fair
Brown	Deep yellow/red		Fashion Fair, Iman, Black Opal
Dark brown/black	Deep yellow/red/blue	Iman	Fashion Fair, Iman, Black Opal

Q&A Session

Q. *My foundation doesn't seem to cover up dark patches on my skin. How do I camouflage skin discolorations?*

A. Many women of color have dark patches or blotches on the skin owing to a variety of causes that include sun damage, skin injury, skin conditions such as acne, certain medications, or underlying medical problems. Your first step should be to uncover the source of the discoloration and try techniques and medications to diminish it, not just cover it up. Visit a dermatologist to determine the source of the problem. The physician may suggest solutions for treating or preventing the underlying problem. Then you can talk with your dermatologist about various ways to lessen dark marks, such as the use of hydroquinone bleaching products or alpha-hydroxy products and peels. You will also need to wear sunscreen daily to protect your skin and speed the fading of dark spots, which may take weeks or months. After the discoloration has been addressed, you should apply concealer a shade lighter than your skin tone to any remaining dark area. If you still have very prominent discolorations, consider products such as Dermablend and Covermark. Then you should make sure your foundation is right for your skin tone and type (see page 18). Don't give in to the temptation to overdo foundation or powder! Dusting powder over one layer of the correct color foundation will give you the complete coverage you seek.

Q. *Is "permanent" makeup safe?*

A. Many salons are offering "permanent" makeup—that is, tattooed eyeliner or lip liner. A technician applies a pigment, using a disposable needle, to the skin of upper or lower eyelids or to the lip line. The advantage is having makeup that does not need to be applied or removed. I rarely recommend permanent makeup because of the potential risks. All tattooing carries the risk of infection. The dyes in the pigment may also cause an allergic reaction. If the lines created are not straight, you're stuck with them. Women of color who have a tendency to develop keloids (raised scars) of course should not get any type of tattoos. You should also be aware that permanent eye lining, though widely available, has not been tested for safety by the Food and Drug Administration.

Q. *My acne gets worse every time I use makeup. How can I avoid flare-ups and still use cosmetics to cover my acne?*

A. If your skin is acne-prone, it requires special care (see chapter 9). The first step is to make sure your acne is being properly treated. If you have not already seen a dermatologist, schedule an appointment. It may take six to eight weeks of treatment to get acne breakouts under control. (If you have acne scars or related discoloration, talk to the dermatologist about the risks and benefits of cosmetic products or procedures to diminish these imperfections.) For acne-prone skin that tends to be oily, you'll need to follow the makeup guidelines for oily skin: after cleansing, wipe away excess oil with toner (if okayed by your dermatologist), use your acne medication and oil-free sunscreen (if needed), and apply a light water-based foundation, followed by translucent powder. Look for products that are labeled "nonacnegenic" or "noncomedogenic." Carry tissue to blot oil during the day and thoroughly remove your makeup at night (but avoid rubbing) to avoid clogged pores and getting makeup on your pillow, where it can end up back on your skin. Be sure to treat acne flare-ups quickly to avoid pigmentation discolorations that can result, and *never* pick at bumps—you'll only aggravate the condition. If problems persist, revisit your dermatologist.

Sunscreen as Makeup?

Sunscreens can help improve the appearance of your skin, especially if you have dark marks or other discolorations. How? First, sunscreens prevent and help speed the fading of dark blotches on the face because they stop UV rays before they can reach the skin and do damage. Also, sunscreens that contain titanium dioxide or zinc oxide tend to impart a white or violet-white hue, which can serve as concealer as well as protection from the sun. (However, sunscreens in makeup do not typically provide enough protection so don't forget to apply sunscreens separately *before* applying makeup.)

Makeup Mistakes Women of Color Make

Here's more advice from makeup artists regarding some common cosmetic blunders.

Don't: Line lips with black eyeliner.

This look, based on a trend set by Naomi Campbell back in the nineties, is no longer in fashion and is not as flattering as some women believe. Lip liner should never look like a dark ring encircling the mouth.

Do: Match lip liner with lipstick and blend.

Your makeup will look more natural if there is no clear line between liner and lipstick. Try colors like plums and burgundies. Or you can blend a neutral tone liner (chestnut, chocolate) with matching lipstick and gloss just in the center. Whatever you do, don't forget to blend.

Don't: Draw in your eyebrows.

To frame the face, some women mistakenly use pencil to create an artificial-looking arch.

Do: Take time to create a natural-looking brow.

Pluck or wax only excess hairs. Enhance thin brows with a combination of light eye pencil strokes—the strokes should look like individual eyebrow hairs. For more definition, add eye shadow matching your brow color.

Don't: Buy foundation a shade lighter or darker than your skin tone.

Many women of color do this consciously to alter their complexion. But it looks obvious.

Do: Select a foundation that blends with your natural tone.

The purpose of foundation is to bring out your natural beauty by evening skin tone. Ask a cosmetics consultant for help in finding the right match and applying it with powder. Once you've learned how to use these products to enhance your beauty, you'll feel better about the skin you're in.

Don't: Forget to blend eye shadow.

Though you may use three different shades of shadow, you should not be able to see the lines between those shades.

Do: Blend, blend, blend.

After you've applied your shadow colors, use a shadow brush, or your fingers, to blend the lines between the colors. The effect will be more flattering and natural.

Don't: Wear too much makeup—or too little.

Some women of color apply too much foundation and powder because they are imitating celebrities or they believe that's how makeup is supposed to look—

thick and cakey. Others, turned off by a "made up" face, wear no makeup at all, or only lipstick.

Do: Wear just enough makeup to bring out your natural beauty.

If you apply concealer and one layer each of foundation and powder, coverage should be complete and even. There's no need for multiple makeup layers. To complete your look, add some complementary eye shadow, mascara, and lipstick. If you've selected the appropriate shades, you will not look too made up—you'll just look like a better you. Consult the experts at a makeup counter for guidance, and take notes.

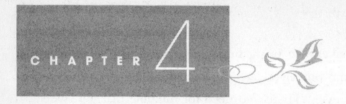

CHAPTER 4

HAIR- AND NAIL-CARE KNOW-HOW

The best way to complement smooth, glowing skin is with a healthy, lustrous head of hair. As a woman of color, you've never before had more hair-care products and styling options at your disposal. Whether you like to wear your hair straight, natural, braided, weaved, with extensions, in cornrows, or in twists—or some combination of these—your hair texture and cultural inheritance make it possible to experiment with a great variety of styles.

But whatever your styling preference, if you're like most women of color, you've probably exposed your hair to harmful and damaging grooming processes. The majority of Black women who I see have hair that is damaged or hair that does not grow the way they would like it to. Many of the styling and processing techniques common among us—chemical relaxers, hot combs, curling irons, and tight braids with extensions and weaves, among others—can take their toll, leaving us with dry, dull, and broken hair. These processes are at least in part responsible for Black women's susceptibility to a long-ignored but serious problem: hair loss and hair breakage.

Like our skin, our hair is distinct from that of White women and requires special care. Among women of color there is a wide range of hair types and textures, so identifying what makes your hair unique is a key step in learning how to care for it. In this chapter you'll learn about the distinctive properties of your hair and how to evaluate your hair's texture and condition. I also discuss what you need to know about washing, conditioning, and styling hair, and I describe hair-care programs for relaxed and natural hairstyles. You'll get clear answers about what causes hair damage and how to avoid it. In chapter 14 we will delve into causes of hair loss and how to treat it.

Finally, this chapter also offers advice on caring for your nails. The risks of popular nail-care practices, such as acrylic nails, are addressed. You'll find out how to determine your nails' health and how to groom them in an attractive, professional way.

BLACK HAIR CHARACTERISTICS

The hair of women of color is in some basic ways like that of White women, but in many other ways it is distinct. The production of all hair starts beneath the skin surface at the base of the hair follicle. Hair is made of the protein keratin, which also occurs in skin. Each hair strand is composed of three layers, including the *cuticle*, or outermost layer, the *cortex* or pigment-producing layer, and the *medulla* or innermost layer. Though keratin is a strong substance and the hair cuticle is designed to resist penetration of excess moisture and chemicals, our hair is by no means indestructible and each layer can be damaged by styling processes we use every day.

Black hair differs from white hair in a number of ways. For example, the follicles of our hair tend to be curved instead of straight. This curvature contributes to the hair's curl. It also contributes to our tendency to develop ingrown hairs after shaving and may even be partly responsible for our propensity for hair loss or alopecia. Because our hair is so tightly coiled, it is often dry since the oil naturally produced in the scalp does not flow down from the curved follicle as readily and does not slide down the curled, knotted hair as it does down a straight follicle and straight hair. That's one reason Black women do not typically need to wash our hair as often

as Whites—our hair simply does not get as oily. So we do not need to wash our hair every day or every other day like women with straight hair. But we do need to wash it more than once a month, which is not the practice of many Black women. Washing weekly is a real must for all Black women. Our grooming practices—relaxing, blow-drying, hot combing, washing once or twice a month—also tend to further dry out our scalps and hair.

Black hair, as seen in cross section under a microscope, tends to have a flat, elliptical shape. A long strand viewed microscopically looks much like a twisted piece of ribbon instead of a straight one. This shape makes the hair more prone to forming very small knots. While this knotting may make it easier to cultivate some styles like locks, it also makes it more difficult to comb and style straightened or natural hair. Because of this tendency, women of color may have more difficulty combing or brushing our hair without pulling on it with excessive force. With constant and forceful combing and brushing comes breakage—a little breakage each day that accumulates. This continuous breakage is why many Black women can't get the length that they desire, falsely believing that their hair won't grow.

Another distinct difference between black and white hair is that Black women have fewer elastic fibers anchoring the hair to the scalp at the dermal layer. With fewer fibers, women of color may be more prone to hair shedding and loss. That characteristic, coupled with our culturally ingrained tendency to pull tightly on hair while braiding, for example, or while gathering hair into a taut ponytail, can lead to problems such as traction alopecia (see chapter 14). The greater number of melanin granules in our hair, which account for its dark color, may also produce free radicals that can cause damage to hair and hair loss.

Black hair has many distinctive properties, but is not, by any means, all the same. Because our heritage often includes Native American, European, and/or Latin ancestry as well as African ancestry, "black hair" comes in endless variations. As a woman of color, you may have hair that is loosely or tightly curled, fine or quite thick, long or short. On your head of hair alone, you may find varying degrees of curl. Hair type, texture, and length are all determined by genes, though some changes may come with age. As you learn about your hair's unique texture

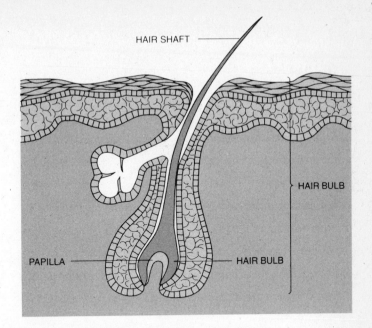

Hair follicle

From Black Skin Care for the Practicing Professional, *1st Edition, by A. P. Thrower and*
H. Gambino, © 1999. Reprinted by permission of Delmar, a division of Thomson Learning.

and condition—and how to work *with* it—you'll be closer to the healthy hair of
your dreams.

TEXTURE AND CONDITION

Understanding your hair's texture and condition will guide you in how to best
wash, condition, and style your hair, and it will help you determine when your
hair has become damaged. Hair texture falls along a spectrum between very fine
and very coarse. Texture is determined by the size of individual hair strands. If a
strand's diameter is small, the hair is fine; strands with a larger diameter are coarse.
To identify your hair's texture, pull a strand from a hairbrush or comb, or right out
of your head, and hold it in one hand between the thumb and forefinger. Then take
the following quiz:

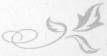

What's My Hair Texture?

1. My hair looks:
   - a. thick
   - b. thin
   - c. in between

2. My hair feels:
   - a. hard
   - b. soft
   - c. in between

3. My hair is:
   - a. wiry
   - b. smooth
   - c. in between

Analysis

- Mostly *a*s: Your hair is medium coarse to coarse.
- Mostly *b*s: Your hair is fine to very fine.
- Mostly *c*s: Your hair has medium texture—between fine and coarse.
- *A, b,* and *c:* Your hair texture falls between medium fine and medium coarse.

Many, but not all, Black women have medium coarse to very coarse hair. A hairstylist can help you further pinpoint your hair's texture, and tell you which hairstyles and products are best for you. For example, women with coarse texture who relax their hair may need a stronger relaxer formula or more contact time while someone with fine hair can use a milder relaxer or texturizer; don't think that coarse hair will allow you to do all sorts of things to it. Coarse hair can also be very delicate. So talk to a licensed stylist to determine what looks best for you.

The Tress Test

The overall condition of your hair is based on three aspects: *porosity*, or its ability to absorb moisture; *elasticity*, or springiness; and *density* (hairs per square inch). Perhaps the most important sign of hair health is elasticity—or lack thereof. To test yours, use the same hair you pulled for the texture quiz (page 80). Hold it now with both hands, between the index fingers and thumbs. Give it a gentle pull. If the hair snaps easily, it has poor elasticity, probably owing to excessive heat from blow-dryers and curling irons or to chemical treatments. If it stretches and springs back, the elasticity is good.

Hair porosity, elasticity, and density should also be assessed by your hairstylist before each treatment. This analysis will help you and her (or him) determine, for example, how much time is required for chemical processes such as hair coloring and chemical relaxing to take effect in your hair, and how well your hair will tolerate such processes. Poor elasticity and frequent breakage are clear signs that your hair has been damaged by styling processes and that you'll need to take better care of it. Don't automatically think that you must have a touch-up every six or eight weeks. Listen to what you hair is telling you. If it is dry and brittle and breaking, then skip the touch-up for six to nine months.

Did You Know?
Healthy hair grows at rate of one-half inch per month.

HAIR CARE AND MAINTENANCE

Because of black hair's tendency to curl, to become dry, to form knots, to break, and to separate from the scalp, our daily grooming practices must be geared more toward protecting the hair than many women of color are used to. This may be difficult considering the popularity of hair relaxers and other harsh heat and chemical processes. But it's not impossible. You can learn to minimize the damage to your hair and still look good. Following are my suggestions for managing relaxed, hot-combed, and natural hair.

Relaxed Hair Care

The majority of Black women—some 75 to 80 percent—chemically relax their hair to make it straight and to wear straight hairstyles. Because of the chemicals used (sodium, lithium, or guanidine hydroxide) to straighten and relax the hair, the relaxed hair of some Black women is fragile and prone to dryness and breakage. Even no-lye relaxers can damage the hair, especially if the directions are not followed explicitly. In fact, many women do not realize that the no-lye preparations may be just as damaging as the lye relaxers. Also potentially damaging are texturizers. Although many women think that texturizers do not contain chemicals, they do. So it's important to think of texturizers as the same as chemical relaxers. Finally, even if your relaxed tresses are in generally good condition, you'll need to treat them gently and condition on an ongoing basis to prevent damage and breakage. And remember that your hair can and does change as time goes on, so always reassess your hair before each chemical process.

One of the biggest mistakes women with chemically relaxed hair make is to get touch-ups too frequently. To straighten new hair growth, many women of color typically get touch-ups every six to eight weeks, or six to nine times a year. To minimize damage to the hair, I recommend a modified schedule—a touch-up every ten to twelve weeks in the winter when there is less humidity and sweat causing new growth to frizz and curl; and every seven to eight weeks in summertime. That adds up to four to five times a year. My reason is simple: the fewer chemical processes you subject your hair to each year, the less damage it will sustain.

There are several important principles to follow when undergoing a touch-up. First, make certain that the chemicals are applied only to the new growth of hair and only by individuals with previous experience. Make sure the stylist uses the strength of hair relaxer most appropriate for your hair type. If your hair is fine or medium coarse, you do not need a "super" strength formula. Do not undergo a touch-up if you have sores or bumps on your scalp. If your scalp itches or if you have been scratching the scalp, postpone the touch-up. Also avoid a touch-up if you have recently dyed or colored your hair. At the hairdresser's, never let the chemical touch the scalp or skin directly. *Do not* allow the stylist to leave the relaxer on for longer than the suggested time—this will only further damage your hair. (Ask the stylist what the directions recommend as the suggested time and do not exceed it.) During the relaxing process, make sure the stylist removes the relaxer at the first sign of scalp tingling. Do not allow the scalp to burn! This is a common practice because many Black women believe that by leaving the relaxer on for as long as they can stand the burning, the hair will be straighter. What they don't realize is that they are inflaming their scalp and hair follicles, which can lead to hair loss. Do not allow the chemical to burn or even tingle moderately—have it washed out at the first sign of mild tingling. Always deep-condition after a touch-up, since the hair is most porous at that time. This way, you will seal the cuticular layer and add shine and manageability to your hair.

Washing. Relaxed hair should be washed every seven to ten days. If your hair is dry or requires elaborate styling, you may be tempted, like many women of color, to wash it infrequently—as little as once or twice a month. However, this can lead not only to dirty hair but to an itchy and flaking scalp, and incredibly dry hair. Unclean hair also tends to look dull and lifeless. Weekly washing will clean the hair of dirt and pollutants as well as the build-up of various products such as hair oils, pomades, gels, and other leave-in products. It also gives you the opportunity to regularly condition your hair.

Select a conditioning shampoo formulated for "chemically treated" hair or for "dry, damaged hair." To wash the hair, wet it thoroughly with warm water and apply a quarter-size amount of shampoo to the scalp. Massage the shampoo throughout the scalp, then squeeze it down through the length of the hair. Rinse completely and shampoo again if needed to remove dirt. Rinse again, making sure no shampoo residue is left in the hair. If you find that you need a dandruff shampoo, and you have relaxed hair, try the following tip. Lather the scalp only (don't squeeze the shampoo down through the length of the hair) and massage the dandruff shampoo into the scalp. Let it stay in contact with the scalp for four to five minutes; rinse. Then wash the entire head, scalp, and hair with your nonmedicated conditioning shampoo.

Conditioning. Regular use of hair conditioners after every shampoo is a must for all black hair, but especially for relaxed hair. Conditioners restore moisture to combat dryness, smooth the cuticle to add shine, and prevent tangling, making the hair more manageable, softer, and easier to style. More manageable hair is less likely to break off and more likely to grow.

You should condition your relaxed hair every seven to ten days with a *deep conditioner* or *reconstructive conditioner*. These typically protein-based conditioning treatments should be combined with heat to penetrate the hair shaft and provide moisture. To condition, squeeze excess water from the hair after you shampoo and rinse. Apply the product and add heat from a hooded hair dryer or warm towel for twenty to thirty minutes or according to product instructions. Make sure to coat the ends, which tend to be the driest part of the hair and most prone to breakage. You may want to gently work the conditioner through the hair with a wide-toothed comb or with your fingers to distribute it evenly. After the required time has passed, thoroughly rinse out the conditioner.

If you have very dry hair, alternate your deep conditioning treatments with *hot-oil treatments* or an *overnight oil treatment*; these products repair damage to the cuticle and restore shine. One strategy is to saturate the hair with the oil at bedtime, cover the entire scalp with a clear shower cap, securing it in place with a scarf, and sleep with the oil on. Wash the oil out with a shampoo for oily hair the next morning and then apply a conditioning shampoo in a second lather. Then condition as directed. Whatever conditioner type you use, be sure to remove all product residue when you rinse. (See "Rx: Hair Reconstruction Regimen," page 260, or www.societyhilldermatology.com.)

Styling. The process of drying and curling relaxed hair often leaves it vulnerable to more damage. To protect your tresses, opt for rollers over curling irons. Curling irons, especially those heated in small electrical units called stoves, become excessively hot. That heat can cause significant damage to the hair. (It also causes those all-too-common curling iron burns on the skin.) The more often you use the curling irons, the more damage will be done. The safest curling irons are thermostatically controlled (plug into the electrical outlet). You should never use curling irons every day for styling. Try to use rollers instead and sit under a hooded hair dryer. Rollers come in various materials, including plastic, tube, and mesh rollers, and give the hair shape and body while keeping it straight. Also exercise caution and care with the use of the new ceramic curling paddles. The excessive heat generated may damage the hair with prolonged use. In general, opt for hood dryers over handheld ones. Handheld dryers can also burn the scalp, hair, and skin—and, of course, damage the hair. If you must use a blow-dryer, go for the medium setting and the lowest wattage it takes to get your hair dry—less than 1,200 watts is safe. Also, hold the dryer about twelve inches away from hair. Apply moisture cream to hair before styling with heat, and by all means, try to minimize the amount and degree of heat applied to relaxed hair.

Another safe way to dry hair and keep it straight is to wrap it tightly around the head, pinning it down with bobby pins. This technique is known as the wrap. You may apply a straightening solution like Aveda's Hair Straightening Lotion. After wrapping the hair, sit under a hooded dryer. When your hair is dry, you may curl just the ends with a warm (not hot) curling iron. Finally, rewrap and cover it up at night with a silk or satin scarf to keep it smooth and untangled.

Trimming. Get your hair trimmed every eight weeks or so to maintain its style and to clip split ends. It's important to have the ends trimmed regularly for the overall health and continued growth of your hair. Finally, if your hair is badly damaged, take the big step and cut off one or two inches to remove all of the broken ends. Then begin your new regimen for achieving and maintaining healthy hair.

Relaxer Lite

If you have curly hair and want to loosen the curl but not completely straighten your tresses, ask your stylist about getting your hair "texturized." Though not as damaging as a full-strength relaxer, texturizers still contain chemicals, so condition your hair regularly to keep it healthy.

Case in Point: Chemical Overkill

Charlotte, a thirty-six-year-old woman who had been using chemical relaxers for twenty years, came to my office complaining about hair loss. When I examined her hair I noticed that her hair length was uneven in areas at the top of the scalp where some strands were only three inches long compared to other areas where the hair was six or seven inches long. Charlotte's hair texture was also dry and brittle, and many of her ends were split and had broken off at the top of the scalp. I asked Charlotte to describe her hair-care routine. She explained that, upon the advice of her hairdresser, she received touch-ups every five to six weeks. In between touch-ups, she visited the hairdresser every two weeks for a wash, blow-dry, and curl. At the salon, her hair was dried with an intensely hot dryer and the hairdresser also used a curling iron heated in a small unit called a stove. At home, Charlotte styled her hair most mornings with an electric curling iron or hot roller set.

My diagnosis? Charlotte's hair breakage was caused by the excess chemicals and heat applied to her hair. I explained to her that her hair's cuticle, or outer layer, and the entire shaft had become weakened and fractured from all the years of processing. All of the hair styling and processes were catching up with her. Charlotte balked when I suggested she stop using relaxers altogether for six to nine months. Instead, we agreed she would cut the number of times she got her hair relaxed in half—from nine times a year to four (in June and August, November, and February). The first step was to have her ends cut and the hair cut to one even length. She would have her hair washed weekly after an overnight oil treatment. Her hairdresser washed her hair twice, applying a shampoo for oily hair to remove the overnight oil and a conditioning shampoo in the second lather, followed by a deep conditioner for twenty minutes. Her hair was then wrapped and dried under a hood dryer. She got trims every six to eight weeks.

By using the deep conditioner, Charlotte kept her "roots"—the new hair grown between relaxers—healthy and manageable. Her hair began to grow without breaking and it became soft and shiny. Six to nine months later, Charlotte had a new head of hair. By minimizing the number of times relaxers were applied to the hair, minimizing the heat applied to her hair, and intensively conditioning her hair on a weekly basis, her hair began to grow.

No Lye

Many women with severely damaged hair continue their touch-ups every six weeks but switch to a "kiddy" perm—relaxers designed for children. This switch usually does not lead to improvement in the damaged hair because the kiddy perm still contains chemicals that cause damage. Instead, women should discontinue the use of the relaxer for a period of time prescribed by a dermatologist.

DRYING TIP

To shorten the amount of time your hair is exposed to heat, towel-dry your hair thoroughly before exposing it to a hair dryer or hood dryer.

Hot-Combed Hair

The hot comb, an alternative tool to straighten thin or coarse hair, is frequently used by Black women when we go to the salon for a "press and curl." But hot combs, like relaxers and hair dryers, can cause damage to the hair and scalp if overused or used improperly. The hot comb itself can reach a very high temperature. The heat from the hot comb can also raise the temperature of pomades used in the straightening process. If the heated oil touches the scalp it can cause burns, and if it seeps into the hair follicle, it can cause inflammation and even hair loss—known as "hot-comb alopecia." This hair loss can, over time, become permanent and quite extensive. Though you probably do not even feel the burn because many of the heated oil droplets are quite small, your hair follicle feels the effect of the heat.

To avoid such damage to the hair and scalp, you must take precautions. Make sure the hair stylist is experienced in the use of hot combs. The hot comb should not be too hot. To test it, your stylist might touch the comb to tissue paper—if the paper browns, the comb is too hot. Most electric combs come with various heat settings, so turn down the heat! If the stylist uses an oven to heat the comb, ask her to minimize the amount of time the comb is left in the oven and allow the comb to cool before applying it to your hair. Once the hair is straight, rollers—not a curling iron—should be used to curl the ends. If you do use a curling iron, make sure it is on a low setting in order to minimize damage to the hair. You should not get your hair hot-combed more than once a week. If your hair is relaxed, I do not recommend using a hot comb on the new growth between touch-ups.

Washing. Hot-combed hair should be washed every seven to ten days. This is particularly important in order to cleanse the hair of pomades and oils used in the straightening process. Select a conditioning shampoo formulated for "dry, damaged hair." Apply a quarter-size amount of shampoo to the scalp. Massage the shampoo throughout the scalp, then squeeze it down to the ends. Rinse completely and shampoo again if needed.

Conditioning. You should condition your hot-combed hair after each shampoo with a *deep conditioner* or *reconstructive conditioner*. To condition, squeeze excess water from hair after shampooing. Apply the product and add heat from a hair dryer or warm towel for twenty to thirty minutes or according to product instructions. Make sure to coat the ends, which tend to be the driest part of the hair. If your hair is especially dry, alternate hot oil treatments with conditioning.

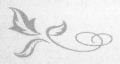

Styling. After the hair has been pressed, you might curl the ends under with a warm—not hot—curling iron. At night, use rollers to maintain the style. Or you can wrap the hair by dividing it into sections, combing in one direction, and pinning it in place around the head. Wear a scarf or hair net to bed. This way, you will wake up with straight hair and no tangles. Do not apply a curling iron in the morning.

Trimming. Get your hair trimmed every eight weeks or so to maintain the style and clip split ends.

HAIR TANGLE TIP

Comb your hair gently with a wide-toothed comb, starting from the ends and working your way up to the roots. Work slowly through knots with your fingers. This will minimize breakage. If hair is especially tangled, use a spray bottle to moisten and loosen knots. Wetting the hair decreases the friction required to comb it.

Protect Your Tresses

In summertime, don't forget that your hair can be damaged by excess sun, salt, and chlorine. At the pool or beach, wrap it in a scarf or wear a sunhat. Wash salt or chlorine out every time you swim.

Natural Hair Care

The term "natural hair" encompasses a wide array of styles, from short naturals to thick Afros, from braids to locks. By natural I mean hair that is not chemically treated, hot-combed, or weaved. The advantage of such styles is that they tend to work with the hair's texture instead of against it, minimizing the potential for damage. They also reflect and proudly display our ethnic heritage. In recent years, these often low-maintenance styles have become more popular and accepted in our

culture and in the mainstream. But don't forget—having a "natural" hairstyle does not mean that you do nothing to your hair.

Washing. Natural hair should be washed once a week. Look for shampoos that contain moisturizers as well as mild cleansers. Products formulated for "dry or damaged" hair may work best. Use a small amount of shampoo to cleanse the scalp and hair strands; rinse thoroughly. Repeat. If you wear braids or cornrows, wash every one to two weeks, paying extra attention to the scalp. Women who wear locks should shampoo weekly or every ten days with products for dry hair.

Conditioning. After shampooing, follow with an *instant conditioner*. Distribute the conditioner throughout the hair, especially on ends, then rinse. If your hair is dry and coarse, treat it to a deep conditioner once a month or so. These treatments will coat the hair shaft and give your natural tresses the shine they need to look healthy and lustrous.

Styling and Trimming. Depending on your style choice, "natural" hair styling may take some time and patience. And you'll still need to be careful not to damage your hair in the process.

Naturals. Whether close-cropped or Afro length, a "natural" cut probably requires the least amount of at-home maintenance. You can air-dry hair or use a low-wattage hair dryer. Use a soft-bristle brush, wide-toothed pick, or your fingers to detangle. A light hair oil or pomade can be used for moisturizing. You may want to also apply a light gel or pomade such as John Paul Mitchell System's Foaming Pomade for styling. You'll need frequent trims—once or twice a month—to maintain the shape of your hair. Wrap hair at night with a silk or satin scarf to prevent frizzing and drying.

Braids/cornrows. To tame frizzing of braids while air-drying, tie a thin scarf around them. Washing regularly is the key to preventing itching and dryness. Individual braids can be worn loose or pulled back in an elegant chignon. You will need to have your hair rebraided every two to twelve weeks. To protect your roots, make sure the hair braider is qualified and experienced. You'll need to make sure she avoids two common mistakes—braiding the hair too tightly and braiding with heavy extensions. Either practice will put stress on your roots and may lead to permanent hair loss. How do you know if the braids are too tight? If you cannot move your forehead or temples or raise your eyebrows after the braids are put in, they are too tight. If you have a headache afterward, they are too tight. Too-tight braiding is responsible for the receding hairlines seen on many Black women who have worn braided styles for years. Wrap hair at night with a silk or satin scarf to prevent frizz and drying.

Locks. Locks take a good deal of work and they are not maintenance-free. You must be committed to their care and have patience. If you use twists to initiate your locks, you will need to retwist hair frequently—several times a month as the new growth appears. To do that, divide just-washed or moistened hair into sections (the smaller the section, the tighter the twist). Divide section in two and twist by either inserting a comb at the ends and turning the comb or by rolling the sections between your palms. Wrap hair at night with a silk or satin scarf to prevent frizz and drying. Variations on locks include yarn locks and silky locks. You will also need to apply a moisturizer, such as Dark and Lovely Tea Tree Oil Lock and Twist Butter or Dark and Lovely Hydrating Citrus Braid and Sheen Spray, to keep locks from getting dry. Don't overtwist or twist too tightly as hair loss could develop. Avoid long, heavy locks, which could lead to hair loss.

Twists. This popular style is a great way to give your hair a rest from chemicals, heat, and styling. Twists are also less permanent than locks and terrifically versatile. From flat twists and two-strand twists to corkscrew twists, you can experiment and find a style that suits your hair texture and length. If you've never had your hair twisted, you might want to go to a salon for a professional twist or you can do it yourself. Avoid pulling on hair to while twisting. Most twist styles last two weeks. Wrap hair at night with a silk or satin scarf to prevent frizzing and unraveling of the style. At the end of the two weeks, take the time to untwist your hair gently to avoid breakage and knotting. Wash with a conditioning shampoo and conditioner. Trim every eight weeks or so. Again, to avoid hair loss or breakage, don't overtwist or twist too tightly.

Summer Hair Repair

Here's a strategy I personally use and call my "summer hair-care repair." During the summer months, I usually wear my hair pulled back in a ponytail or chignon. At the beginning of the summer I have my ends trimmed to remove split and broken hairs. I then wash my hair weekly with a conditioning shampoo, and apply a conditioner for dry and damaged hair evenly throughout my hair. I leave the conditioner in my hair without rinsing it out. Then I comb my hair, towel dry, pull it back, and go. The conditioning and minimal styling gives my hair a healthy reprieve. By the end of the summer (without heat, chemicals, or blow-drying) my hair is healthy—no split ends—and shiny.

Case in Point: Getting Hair to Grow

Keisha, age twenty-five, came to me with the complaint that her hair simply would not grow. She asked me to run blood tests to determine whether she might have a vitamin deficiency or hormonal imbalance. But besides her poor hair growth, Keisha was otherwise healthy. In fact, she took a multi-vitamin each day and ate a balanced diet. The real source of her problem was her hair-care routine. Because her hair was short, and new growth is more obvious in short hair, Keisha had her hair relaxed every four weeks. She also had highlights and used a curling iron every morning for styling. Upon my advice, Keisha decided to give up relaxers to get the hair growth she wanted. She chose to wear braids instead. To prevent further hair damage, she made sure the hair braider used natural hair braided very loosely. She also used extensions that were less than shoulder length. With loose braids and short extensions, she avoided excessive tension on the hair follicle. Keisha agreed to wash and condition her hair every ten days and have her braids redone every ten weeks. After nine months of this regimen, she could see a real difference in the length of her hair.

Myth: Brushing hair with a hundred strokes a day will keep it shiny and healthy.
Fact: The logic behind this fallacy is based on the idea that brushing hair brings the natural oils from the roots to the ends. But a hundred strokes may just pull out a hundred hairs! Women of color, who are more prone to hair tangling and hair loss, can keep hair soft and shiny with regular conditioning treatments.

Must-Have Hair Tools
To avoid breakage, make sure your hair-care tools are gentle and in good shape. Avoid plastic or cheaply made products, which can catch and pull out hair. What you need:
   Wide-toothed comb
   Natural bristle brush
   Hairpins of varying sizes
   Ponytail holders, made of satin or silk
   Scarf, made of satin or silk
   Shower cap
   Rollers (mesh, tubes)
   Spray bottle

Dealing with Dandruff

Black women may be prone to developing dry, itching scalps because we tend to wash our hair infrequently (every three to four weeks) and dry the scalp with heat from blow-dryers and hot combs. Residues from gels, mousses, and hair sprays can also build up and cause itching. Greasing the scalp will not solve this problem. To control the flaking, it's best to wash your hair more frequently—at least once a week. If you indeed have dandruff, which tends to worsen in winter, try a medicated shampoo such as T Gel Shampoo by Neutrogena, Head and Shoulders, or Nizoral Shampoo. To avoid drying out the hair with these products, lather the scalp only and massage the dandruff shampoo into the scalp for no longer than four to five minutes. After shampooing, use a conditioning shampoo and deep conditioning treatment for ten to twenty minutes. You may also want to try nonmedicated shampoos that contain tea tree oil (Paul Mitchell's Tea Tree Shampoo), a natural ingredient that fights flaking without excessive drying.

If, however, frequent washing does not get dandruff under control—and if it migrates to your eyebrows and face—you may have an underlying condition that needs to be treated. See your dermatologist.

Pomade and Pimples

Hair pomades or hair oils—containing various mixtures of petroleum, lanolin, and oils—may do wonders for enhancing the manageability of our hair, but they can wreak havoc on our skin. These products often spread to the forehead and temples, producing acne pimples. To avoid this problem, only use pomades if you need them. Opt for the lightest pomades you can find (Aveda Pure-Fume Brilliant Humectant Pomade or Modern Elixirs' Defining Pomade). Apply them lightly and away from the hairline and temples.

A Word About Weaves

Hair weaving—the process of adding synthetic or human hair to natural hair—can create the illusion of fullness and length. With weaves, you can grow out a short cut or experiment with different styles that you may not be able to achieve with your natural hair alone. A hairstylist can add a weave to your hair by either braiding in extensions, sewing hair onto cornrowed hair, or bonding (gluing) hair to your natural hair strands at the root. It's easier to use human hair, which you can wash and condition like your own hair, but human hair is more expensive than synthetic strands. Synthetic strands can be itchy and scratchy and don't blend in as well with your natural hair.

Weaves do have a downside. The adhesives used in the bonding methods can irritate the skin and scalp and produce a rash. When removing the bonded hair, some of your natural hair can be inadvertently pulled out as well (and you want to hold on to every one of your hairs). Many women avoid washing their hair when their weave is bonded, but this is not a good practice. Even if the process has to be done every two weeks, you must wash your hair.

With a braided weave, too much added hair can weigh down your natural hair, pull at the roots, and weaken the hair, causing hair loss. This is a real concern for women of color whose hair may not be as securely anchored to the scalp. For that reason, you should forgo very long weaves. Weaving is also a long process, taking up to eight hours in some cases depending upon how many tracts you have. To get a good weave, you'll need to select a stylist who has a lot of experience with weaved hair. The stylist should know not only how to minimize stress to the hair and scalp but how to properly match the color and texture of weaved hair to your natural hair for a realistic, seamless look.

Once the weave is in, don't forget to wash and condition it once a week. You'll need to return to the stylist to have the weave tightened every six to eight weeks. The weave should last about four months.

IN LIVING COLOR

It seems more and more women of color are using hair dye not just to cover gray but also to enhance their appearance. Hair coloring can add depth and volume to the hair—not to mention richness to your complexion. You can try highlights for a subtle contrast or a whole new color. The number of shades available today is truly endless.

For the most natural look and least time-consuming process, choose a color one shade lighter or one shade darker than your natural color. Black hair color tends to run from medium brown to black, so the best shades for us range from honey to cinnamon to chocolate. Some auburns and burgundies can also be flattering complements. Lighter shades like blonde require a longer process and more upkeep, especially if you have very dark black hair.

To color your hair safely, do not relax the hair at the same time. The multiple chemical processes can result in hair that is dry, brittle, and prone to breakage. If you have relaxed hair, it is safest to use a color rinse similar to your natural color; do not use permanent hair color to lighten the hair. Also, if you have never colored your hair before, be aware that Blacks have an increased sensitivity to para-phenylenediamine, an ingredient in dark brown and black hair dyes. The dyes can cause an allergic reaction manifested by redness, swelling, and itching of the scalp, eyes, and face. If this occurs, you won't be able to use brown and Black dyes in the future. Be sure to first test the dye on your skin each time you use it, since allergies can develop at any time.

Hair coloring is performed through one of three processes: temporary coloring (rinses), semi-permanent coloring, and permanent coloring. Permanent coloring, which involves the use of chemicals to strip the natural color before adding the new one, will result in the most dramatic and long-lasting color changes. It is also most likely to cause damage. Whatever process you use, be sure to condition the hair weekly to fortify it. Color-enhancing shampoos and conditioners, like Redken Color Extend Shampoo and Conditioner, will help make semi-permanent color last longer. You might also want to apply daily leave-in conditioners like Soft Sheen Breakthru Everyday Moisturizing Lotion. (See the Hair Color Chart for more guidance on hair color.)

HAIR COLOR CHART

PROCESS	RESULT	RISKS	MAINTENANCE
Temporary coloring (*rinse*)	Enhances natural color; covers gray	Minimal	Repeat with each shampoo
Semi-permanent	Enhances natural color; darkens color; adds shine	Minimal	Protect color with color-enhancing shampoo, conditioner; repeat in six to twelve weeks
Permanent	Lightens or darkens color several shades; covers gray	Weakens hair; may cause allergic reaction to dye; do not use on recently relaxed hair	Condition weekly with deep penetrating product; touch up in six to twelve weeks

Henna Hints

Though henna, derived from the dry leaves of the *Lawsonia alba* shrub, is a natural hair dye, it's not necessarily benign. Whether applied to the hair for reddish highlights or to the hands for decoration, natural or compound henna can cause allergic reactions and even contact dermatitis in susceptible people. (Wash the area several times and take an antihistamine if this occurs.) Always test on a small area of skin before using.

At-Home Hair Care?

To minimize the cost of hair care, many women may opt to relax and color their hair at home. However, I don't recommend this unless you've already had lots of experience with the use of these chemicals and do not have damaged hair. To avoid damaging your tresses, it's worth it to see a licensed and experienced hair stylist.

Repairing Damaged Hair

If your hair has been noticeably damaged (split ends, breakage) by chemical processes or too much heat, take these steps to repair it:

1. Stop using chemical relaxers, hair dyes, blow-dryers, curling irons, and hot combs for at least six to nine months.
2. Wash and condition hair weekly. Use deep penetrating or restructuring conditioners each week and alternate with hot oil treatments if your hair is especially dry.
3. Dry hair without excessive heat either by air-drying or wrapping it before going under a warm hood dryer.
4. Get trims every six to eight weeks.
5. If you must, resume relaxers or hair coloring on a less frequent schedule—no more than five times a year.

(For severely damaged hair, see "Rx: Hair Reconstruction Regimen," page 260.)

The Dermatologist's Hair-Care Routine

You may be wondering how, as a dermatologist and woman of color, I keep my relaxed hair healthy. Here's my routine: I wash and condition my hair each week, leaving the conditioner in for ten minutes. I have my hair relaxed by a licensed hairdresser every ten to fourteen weeks, making sure the stylist washes the relaxer out at the first sign of tingling. (I never let it get to the point where it burns.) Afterward, I ask to have my hair set in rollers and dried under a dryer—no blow dryers or curling irons allowed on a regular basis. At night, I sleep in rollers or use pin curls. Every twelve weeks or so, I have my hair trimmed and once or twice a year, I also get highlights but never right before or after a relaxer treatment. To keep the highlights from drying out my hair, I give it extra conditioning. To minimize any breakage, I avoid excessive combing or brushing. In summer, when I swim, I wear my hair pulled back, which means less wear and tear. I always wash the chlorine out after swimming and leave a small amount of conditioner in. My philosophy is, the less done to your hair, the better its condition will be.

NAILING IT

Neat, well-groomed nails put the finishing touch on our appearance. These days, professional women opt for anything from lengthy polished nails to short nails with clear polish. Either way can look sharp. But some nail trends popular among women of color, such as extra-long tips or acrylic nails, carry risks. Also, since our nails may have discolorations that are normal (a brown streak on each nail), and others that are not (a streak on one nail only, which may indicate cancer), we need to be particularly mindful of our nail health.

Our nails, like our hair, are made of keratin. The nail plate, which contains no nerves or blood vessels, lies atop the nail bed, which has a blood supply (see illustration, page 100). Our nails tend to grow slowly, just a couple of millimeters per month, but that rate of growth can vary slightly from nail to nail and during different periods in our lives such as pregnancy. The health of our nails is determined by many factors, including our diet and our overall health, as well as our nail-care practices.

Nail Do's and Don'ts

Don't: Wear acrylic nails.

One of the most common problems I see is with the use of acrylic nails—artificial nails attached over the nail plate with a chemical adhesive. This type of artificial nail is stronger and lasts longer than plastic preformed nails. But they can lead to thinning of your natural nail and promote the growth of bacteria or fungus in your nails. The signs of a fungal infection are yellow or opaque nails, nails that are lifted off of the underlying nail bed, and twisted nails. Bacterial infections may turn the nail green or cause the cuticle area to become red and

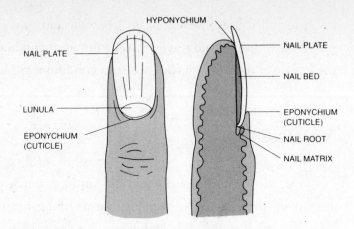

Nail structure

From Black Skin Care for the Practicing Professional, *1st Edition, by A. P. Thrower and*
H. Gambino, © 1999. Reprinted with permission of Delmar, a division of Thomson Learning.

swollen. If you see signs of infection, visit your doctor immediately. Fungal infections of the fingernails can be treated with an oral medication that is taken for
six weeks (there are several potentially serious side effects that you must discuss
with your doctor) or with a topical nail lacquer (requires many months of daily
application before you see an improvement). Another reason to ditch acrylics is
that the chemical adhesive can also trigger an allergic reaction. Finally, if you
can't give up the acrylics permanently, consider giving your nails a break by stopping the use of the acrylics during the summer since the heat and humidity of
the sun help promote the growth of fungus and bacteria.

Do: Encourage natural nail growth by protecting your nails from harsh soaps and
cold weather, moisturizing your hands daily, clipping and gently filing the nails
regularly, and giving your nails a break from drying polish and removers that
contain acetone.

Don't: Cut your cuticles.

Though cutting the cuticles at the base of the nail plate can make fingernails and
toenails appear more neat and flawless, it frequently causes problems. Removal
of the cuticle can promote bacterial and yeast infections. If you bleed during a

manicure or pedicure, you also potentially expose yourself to the transmission of diseases such as hepatitis and HIV.

Do: Ask your manicurist to simply push back the cuticle to give it a neat appearance. You can also keep cuticles tamed by wearing gloves when you wash dishes and in cold weather, and by moisturizing your hands several times daily.

Don't: Grow extra-long nails.

Nails that grow farther than an inch away from the fingers may be eye-catching but they can also be troublesome. Long nails are more readily damaged during the course of the day. They can also harbor fungus and bacteria if not kept thoroughly cleaned underneath. These lengthy tips make it more difficult to perform daily activities and care for your hair and skin.

Do: Opt for a more professional-looking, slightly shorter nail. Regular at-home or in-salon manicures will keep them looking sharp.

Basic Nail Care

Don't ignore your nails between manicures and special occasions. For strong, healthy-looking nails, you need to follow a nail-care program. To keep your tips in tip-top shape:

- Protect your hands and nails from harsh soaps and extreme weather. Use mild soap to wash your hands and wear gloves in winter.
- Moisturize your hands daily with a creamy lotion. Be sure to work lotion into the cuticles. Carry a pocket-size moisturizer in your purse.
- Keep nails clipped short. File them in one direction only to create an even nail shape and to avoid nail breakage. Don't forget to clean under the nail.
- Take regular breaks from nail polish, which dries the nails. Buff nails for shine.
- Optional: Get a manicure once a month or so. If you get a professional manicure, check to see that the salon and technicians are licensed. Also, take note of whether the facilities and tools are kept disinfected and sterilized.

At-Home Manicure

How to do it yourself:

1. Remove old polish with nonacetone remover and a cotton ball.
2. Gently file nails in one direction only and under the nail to create a smooth, rounded shape.
3. Soak hands in warm sudsy water for five minutes.
4. Pat dry; apply a cuticle softener and push back cuticles with a nail stick wrapped in cotton.
5. Snip hangnails *carefully* with nail scissor or clipper. Or simply smooth them with moisturizer until they shed naturally. Don't clip your cuticle.
6. Moisturize and massage hands with a rich creamy lotion; wipe off excess with a warm, damp cloth.
7. Apply a base coat layer of polish, starting with a stroke down the middle, then on either side. Let dry.
8. Apply one coat of polish from cuticle to tip; let dry; apply the second coat. Choose a color that matches your makeup or clothes.
9. Allow nails twenty minutes to dry completely.

Signs of Poor Nail Health
- Yellow or opaque nails
- White spots on nails or cuticle
- Thick, brittle, or twisted nails
- Pale nail beds
- Red, painful cuticles
- Nail separation

If you even suspect your unhealthy nails may be telling you something, see your doctor or a dermatologist right away. Be sure to note any other symptoms you might have and any recent changes in your diet or lifestyle.

A POLISHED, PROFESSIONAL YOU

Many women of color experiment with intricate hair and nail designs that often take hours to arrange and maintain. But some of these styles—elaborate hairdos and decorative nails—may be less than ideal for hair and nail health, not to mention quite expensive. Unless you are a model or work in a salon, these fashions also are often not appropriate for the workplace. If you enjoy wearing, say, a fancy updo that requires lots of curling iron heat, or acrylic nails with complex designs, consider only wearing them on special occasions—a party, long weekend, or vacation. This way you can still indulge in styles you like but limit the amount of damage they do, such as hair breakage and permanent nail thinning.

You can also save time and money and simplify your beauty routine by going low-maintenance. Opt for short to medium-length nails, which are appropriate for any work environment. Wear your hair pulled back or in a bun to give it a break from the wear and tear of styling. This eliminates the constant need for hot curlers, curling irons, and frequent touch-ups. You can also try braids with short to medium-length extensions, or neat locks, worn down or in a ponytail for a professional appearance. By taking a low-maintenance, professional approach for every day, you save your hair and nails from the effects of damaging processes. In the long run, you'll be more beautiful because your hair and nails will look and feel stronger and healthier.

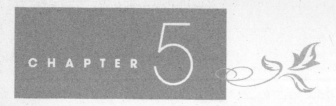

CHAPTER 5

PEELS, LASERS, AND MORE: HIGH-TECH SKIN CARE

While following your daily skin-care program can improve your appearance and help give you the smooth, clear complexion you desire, you may still have skin-care concerns that a basic at-home program doesn't resolve. In that case, you may need the aid of additional products, dermatological treatments, or procedures to look your best. Women of color who have persistent blackheads, dark spots, and acne or chicken pox scars can benefit from a number of new and older "high-tech" techniques. However, because of the sensitive nature of our melanin, we must be particularly careful in choosing procedures and avoiding those that can potentially cause damage to our skin. If you are prone to skin discolorations and keloids, you need to be especially aware of the risks.

You've probably heard or read about such skin rejuvenation techniques as chemical peels, laser treatments, and microdermabrasion, among others. Perhaps you've experimented with one or more of these procedures. In this chapter, you'll learn about the benefit of many popular high-tech skin therapies and techniques and the specific risks for women of color, in addition to the costs and other factors that'll help you decide whether a procedure may be for you. A chart at the end of the chapter provides this information at a glance. You'll learn how to select a skilled practitioner and what questions to ask. I'll also briefly describe some popular cosmetic surgeries and what you need to know about them.

HIGH-TECH AT HOME

Before seeking professional treatments, you can try to take your beauty routine to the next level with over-the-counter or prescription products that you can apply at home. These at-home agents are often used in conjunction with in-office treatments but can be useful on their own. They include the following.

Amazing Acids (Alphahydroxy, Betahydroxy Acids)

These naturally occurring compounds provide a wide range of good-skin benefits. Cleansers, creams, and lotions containing alphahydroxy acids (AHAs) or betahydroxy acids (BHAs) help to exfoliate the outer layer of skin and unclog pores while enhancing elasticity and firmness. They also trap water to moisturize skin. Topical AHA products are available in a range of strengths. Some lotions contain only 5 percent glycolic acid, for example, and other products contain as much as 20 percent. Whether you have dry, oily, or combination skin, cleansing or moisturizing with products containing glycolic acid (an AHA) or salicylic acid (a BHA) will give you a clearer, smoother complexion.

I tend to favor the AHA-containing products, such as the MD Forte or Neostrata products, for most people. BHAs usually work well on oily, acne-prone skin. Women also experience fewer problems such as burning and tingling with BHAs (several Clinique products contain BHAs). Regular use of hydroxy acid products may help diminish discolorations caused by hyperpigmentation. However, some women experience dryness or skin irritation. If you have sensitive skin, test the product on a small area of unexposed skin before applying it to your face. If you have a reaction such as redness or burning sensation within a day or so, switch to a product with a lower concentration of hydroxy acid, one with polyhydroxy acids, or discontinue use altogether. Don't neglect the sunscreen; hydroxy acid products can make the skin more sensitive to sun exposure.

Vitamins A–Z

The vitamins we need in our bodies can be beneficial when absorbed in the skin as well. Products that contain vitamins or vitamin derivatives may help improve our complexions in a number of ways. At the very least, the antioxidant vitamins (C and E) may protect and add moisture to the skin. But be careful not to "OD" on these vitamin-containing skin products—many claimed benefits have yet to be confirmed by reliable scientific research. The vitamins also often break down and lose their efficacy over time.

A Is for Acne and Anti-Aging. Vitamin A is an antioxidant that helps prevent and reverse damage caused by free radicals—harmful molecules that form in the skin when it is exposed to ultraviolet light. Those molecules, which damage DNA, are responsible for the common signs of aging—fine lines, wrinkles, sun spots, skin sagging. Over-the-counter products containing vitamin A derivatives, such as retinol or retinoic acid, help prevent and even reverse sun damage by remodeling and re-forming the collagen-building blocks of the skin, which keep the skin firm and elastic. Prescription products derived from vitamin A (Retin-A, Differin, Tazorac, Avita) provide additional benefits such as clearing acne, unclogging pores, and smoothing the complexion. They are most effective for improving collagen as compared to the over-the-counter products. Over-the-counter products include RoC Retinol Actif Pur Anti-Wrinkle Treatment and Avon Anew Line Eliminator Dual Retinol Facial Treatment. The downside is that vitamin A products can be drying and irritating. Preparations with low concentrations of the vitamin's derivatives may be preferable.

C Is for Cancer Prevention. Another antioxidant, vitamin C helps control free radicals and reduce the sun damage that can lead to skin cancer. It does not, however, diminish wrinkles, smooth the skin, or act as a sunscreen. Topical vitamin C can be applied directly to the skin in the form of creams, patches, or serums. Products to try are Cellex-C High Potency Serum and Lather Vitamin C Facial Serum. Vitamin C can also be found in moisturizers, sunscreens, and eye creams. Because vitamin C can degrade and become ineffective quite easily, however, it should be stored away from sunlight and not combined with vitamin A or hydroxy acids.

E Is for Extra Protection. Vitamin E can provide more antioxidant protection and enhance the effects of vitamin C. But more research is needed to determine just how effective this vitamin is in topical form.

K Is for Clotting. This vitamin may lessen bruising and dark under-eye circles caused by poor blood clotting. Though the efficacy of topical vitamin K is still being debated, studies have shown a benefit. Contrary to rumor, it does not treat broken blood vessels. You can find this vitamin in certain moisturizers, eye creams, and sunscreens.

Lightening Up

Bleaching agents or skin lighteners are useful for restoring an even tone to blotchy, discolored skin. They can also reduce the appearance of freckles. A widely used skin lightener, hydroquinone, is found in both over-the-counter and prescription products that may contain additional ingredients to improve the skin. Hydroquinone works by stopping the overproduction of melanin that causes skin discoloration in the first place. Patch-test on a small area of the skin first since some people are allergic to hydroquinones.

If an over-the-counter preparation containing 2 percent hydroquinone does not achieve the effect you desire, consult a dermatologist for a stronger product. Dermatologists can prescribe 4 percent products, which are frequently more effective. It's important to also use sunscreen year-round and to treat your skin gently to prevent further discoloration. Lightening products should be used only to help even out skin tone within a six-month period. The only potential side effect from prolonged use is a condition called exogenous ochronosis or a paradoxical darkening of the skin. No one knows why this occurs. This reaction to hydroquinone is more common in Africa but does occur in the United States. The only treatment is discontinued use of the product.

Case in Point: Bleaching Away Blotches

When Carol, twenty-two, first came to my office, she had several bumps on her forehead, cheeks, and chin owing to a moderately severe acne problem. I prescribed acne medications and over the next eight weeks nearly all of the bumps on her face were eliminated. But during her next visit Carol came close to tears because she felt her complexion had not improved. She believed that some dark marks that remained on her skin were acne. In fact, the marks were the result of postinflammatory hyperpigmentation, or a darkening of the skin that can occur as a result of acne breakouts.

To treat Carol's dark marks, I prescribed a topical product containing hydroquinone (a bleaching agent), glycolic acid (an alphahydroxy acid exfoliant), and sunscreen. She applied the product twice a day for eight weeks. Upon her next visit, I noticed her dark marks were fading nicely. For the first time since I'd met Carol, she was holding her head high and making eye contact. By the end of her fourth visit, when I told Carol how pretty she looked, her once acne-ridden face beamed.

THE APPEAL OF PEELS

Facial peels can improve your complexion by providing deep exfoliation, which is the removal of the outer layer of skin, revealing the new, smooth, and clear skin underneath. Peels can unclog pores, reduce the appearance of scars, and minimize wrinkles. An older generation of peels, known as trichloracetic acid peels, achieves its effects by using a very strong chemical to penetrate deeply into the skin. This type of peel, however, has many potentially negative side effects and should be used very carefully by women of color and only administered by very experienced hands.

The newer, more popular peels, including alphahydroxy acid (AHA) peels and betahydroxy acid (BHA) peels, provide a more superficial but effective exfoliation. They may also stimulate the production of collagen, a protein that helps preserve skin elasticity and firmness. If you have mild skin discoloration, a series of peels can literally help unveil a more clear, even complexion and radiant skin. These peels may be the best option for most women of color since they remove only the uppermost layers of skin, avoiding the risk of scarring or darkening caused by hyperpigmentation.

Another procedure that has similar benefits as the superficial peels is microdermabrasion. Gentler than traditional dermabrasion, microdermabrasion involves the use of a machine that exfoliates the uppermost layer of the skin using suction and fine crystals.

There are three forms of high-tech exfoliation that remove deeper layers of the skin, providing greater benefits than either hydroxy acid peels or microdermabrasion (but also with potentially greater risks). These procedures are dermabrasion and deeply resurfacing peels, including TCA and Obagi (blue peels). You should consider these stronger procedures only if AHA or BHA peels or microdermabrasion are not effective, or if you are trying to treat deep scars or wrinkling. The descriptions that follow will help you understand the pros and cons of popular peels (approximate costs are based on a survey conducted by the American Society of Dermatologic Surgery).

Hydroxy Acid Peels (Alphahydroxy Acid, Betahydroxy Acid)

- **What it is:** A facial treatment that uses a naturally occurring acid (glycolic acid, fruit acid, salicylic acid) combined with other skin-care ingredients to peel off the uppermost layer of skin. You can receive a low-concentration peel (20 percent hydroxy acid or less) at a spa or salon; higher-concentration peels should be delivered by physicians. Of the two, the betahydroxy acid peel is slightly more effective. It is also better for oily skin because it decreases the oil. (See page 38 for guidance in selecting a spa professional.)

- **Benefits:** Fading of dark spots caused by hyperpigmentation or melasma; unclogged pores; reduction of fine lines; some improvement of dark under-eye circles; improvement in acne; smooth, clear complexion. Slight improvement of acne scars.
- **Risks:** Tingling or burning in skin; dry skin, redness, or peeling after treatment. If you have sensitive skin, ask about the more gentle amino fruit acid facial peels or begin with a very low concentration (less than 20 percent) of the peel products.
- **Cost:** Approx. $600–$900 for six treatments.
- **Recovery time:** None.
- **Maintenance:** At-home use of creams containing AHAs or BHAs beginning at least a week after treatment. Consult your spa professional or physician.

The Obagi Nu-Derm System (Blue Peel)

- **What it is:** A medium-strength facial peel that involves the use of exfoliating acids, skin bleaching agents, and other ingredients to penetrate and remove the skin's uppermost surfaces. The depth of the peel depends on the number of passes or layers applied. This procedure is performed in a doctor's office with or without anesthesia.
- **Benefits:** Improvement of fine lines and deeper wrinkles; reduction in sun damage and dark spots; smooth, even skin tone.
- **Risks:** Dryness, redness, itching, further skin discoloration, burning. Temporary worsening of acne or wrinkles.
- **Cost:** Up to $1,000 per peel.
- **Recovery time:** One week; results peak after six weeks and fade over time.

- *Maintenance:* At-home application of Obagi products, including an exfoliant, skin-bleaching agent, eye cream and sunscreen, beginning after healing.

Trichloracetic acid (TCA)

- *What it is:* A medium-depth facial peel that involves the use of a strong acid to penetrate and remove the skin's outer surface. The procedure is performed in a doctor's office with or without anesthesia.
- *Benefits:* Reduction in acne scars, improvement of fine lines and deeper wrinkles; removal of sun damage and dark spots.
- *Risks:* Possible scarring and further skin discoloration.
- *Cost:* Approx. $950 per treatment.
- *Recovery time:* One week.
- *Maintenance:* Topical cream containing alphahydroxy acid, vitamin A derivatives, and sunscreen beginning after healing.

Microdermabrasion

- *What it is:* A nonchemical treatment that provides a slightly deeper exfoliation than AHA or BHA facials. A machine first sprays a layer of fine aluminum oxide crystals over the skin, then vacuums the crystals, exfoliating the outer layer of skin. This procedure is performed in a doctor's office.
- *Benefits:* Fading of minor dark spots; unclogged pores and removal of blackheads; reduction in acne and other (nonkeloid) scars; lessening of fine lines; smooth, clear complexion.
- *Risks:* Redness; infection; scarring; darkening or lightening of skin.
- *Cost:* $150–$300 per treatment, for up to six sessions.
- *Recovery time:* None.
- *Maintenance:* Topical preparations containing either AHAs or vitamin A derivatives and sunscreen after treatment is completed.

Dermabrasion

- *What it is:* A treatment that uses a special machine to remove the entire outer layer of skin, or the epidermis. It more deeply penetrates the skin to correct significant problems. The procedure is performed in a doctor's office with anesthesia.
- *Benefits:* Reduction in acne and other (nonkeloid) scars; fading of dark spots; unclogged pores and removal of blackheads; lessening of fine lines and deep wrinkles.
- *Risks:* Pain; redness; infection; scarring; darkening or lightening of skin.
- *Cost:* $1,300–$1,500 per treatment.
- *Recovery time:* Two weeks.
- *Maintenance:* Topical preparations containing AHAs, vitamin A derivatives, and sunscreen beginning after healing.

ANCIENT AFRICAN SKIN CARE

Cleopatra's famous milk baths were an early form of sophisticated skin care. Milk contains lactic acid, an alphahydroxy acid that exfoliates and revitalizes the skin.

Case in Point: The Power of Peels

When Jocelyn, a fifty-five-year-old African-American woman, came to see me, she was concerned about a dull and uneven skin tone. Her goal was simple: to have a more radiant, glowing complexion and feel better about herself. After examining her skin, I assessed that she did indeed have darkened skin tones that were not completely even and that her skin was slightly ashen and rough to the touch. This was most likely due to sticky skin cells and a lack of exfoliation. My prescription for Jocelyn included a combination of exfoliating treatments to gently fade the discoloration and restore uniformity to her skin tone. Her treatment regimen consisted of a glycolic acid cleanser and day cream, a more intensive glycolic acid night cream, and a series of six glycolic acid peels, one every three to four weeks.

After the first two peels Jocelyn was discouraged because she did not immediately notice a difference in her skin. But after the third and fourth peels, she began to see her complexion transform from dull and ashy to glowing, smooth, and soft. Her newly radiant skin was soon matched by an even more radiant smile. To maintain her revitalized look, Jocelyn returns to my office every six months for a touch-up peel. She also maintains the use of the glycolic cleanser and day and night creams.

THE LOWDOWN ON LASERS

Ever wish you could zap away certain skin problems? It's possible with the development of laser technology, which can be used to treat a variety of skin conditions, from (nonkeloid) scars to broken blood vessels and warts. Lasers are useful because they enable the practitioner to target specific facial areas and damaged skin layers, while limiting the potential harm to skin. But there are risks. Laser treatments can cause inflammation, damage cells, and, in the hands of an unskilled practitioner, cause injury. If damaged, skin of color is more likely to become scarred or discolored.

Before you consider any type of laser treatment, it's important to make sure it's the best option for your skin condition. You'll need to find a qualified physician with knowledge and experience treating skin of color (see "Questions to Ask the Doctor," page 114). Here's what you need to know about popular laser procedures.

Laser Resurfacing

- **What it is:** A treatment involving the use of laser beams (either Erbium:YAG or CO_2 lasers) on the outer layers of skin. Resurfacing is performed under local or general anesthesia in a doctor's office.
- **Benefits:** Lessens moderate to severe scarring (acne, chicken pox); diminishes

dark spots caused by hyperpigmentation; improves fine lines; tightens skin and rejuvenates complexion.

- **Risks:** Infection, scarring or dark patches, and other pigmentation problems.
- **Cost:** $2,000–$2,400.
- **Recovery time:** One to two weeks with Erbium; two weeks or more with CO2.
- **Maintenance:** After healing is complete, daily use of alphahydroxy acid containing cleanser and lotion in the morning, and a Retin-A or retinol product at night. Sunscreen.

Pulsed Dye and Other Lasers

- **What it is:** Laser technologies that use beams to eliminate or reduce the appearance of broken blood vessels, spider veins, birthmarks, stretch marks, (nonkeloid) scars, and tattoos. (Lasers for hair removal are discussed in Chapter 14.) These include the Pulsed-Dye Laser, Argon Laser, Krypton Laser, Versa-Pulse Laser, and Nlite Laser, among others.
- **Benefits:** Lasers effectively remove unsightly broken blood vessels or spider veins without risk of scabbing or infection.
- **Risks:** Inflammation, redness. Possible bruising, scarring, and hyperpigmentation of the skin.
- **Cost:** $200–$1,500, depending on laser and size of treatment area.
- **Recovery time:** One to two weeks depending on procedure; consult physician.
- **Maintenance:** Broken blood vessels may reappear and require repeated treatment.

Questions to Ask the Doctor

For the best results with any cosmetic procedure, you'll need a skilled physician with extensive experience. To find a doctor, ask for referrals from your family practitioner or friends. You may want to speak to two or three physicians before choosing one. It may be preferable to work with a physician of color or one who is knowledgeable about skin of color. Don't forget that it's important for you to feel comfortable with the practitioner and his or her staff. Before you make an appointment, schedule a consultation and pose questions such as:

What are your credentials?

Do you have training in cosmetic surgery and this procedure in particular?

How many procedures of this kind have you performed?

How many of those procedures were on people of color?

What results can I expect?

What are the risks of this procedure?

Can I see before-and-after pictures?

Can I speak to your previous patients?

How long is the recovery period?

What if the procedure doesn't achieve the result I want?

More Than a Pretty Face

Skin rejuvenation advances such as facial peels, resurfacing, and dermabrasion can erase fine lines, freckles, and scars from your neck, chest, and hands, as well as your face.

Q&A Session

Q. *What are skin tags and how can I get rid of them?*

A. The small brown growths that appear on the face and neck of many people of color are often referred to as skin tags or *dermatosis papulosa nigra*. Some people believe that removal of the growths will cause excessive bleeding or, worse, cancer. Relatives and friends, particularly those from the South, may tell stories of tying string around the growths, causing them to fall off.

The truth is that skin tags are natural overgrowths of skin that are benign. Skin tags may be more likely to develop during pregnancy and as you age. They may appear under the arms or breasts or in the groin. The tendency to get these growths is inherited. They will not fall off or disappear with the use of creams or lotions. Most important, they will not become cancerous. However, if you want to remove them, do it safely. A dermatologist can snip off the growths surgically or cauterize (burn) them. Cauterization involves the application of an electric needle to the area, which burns the growth, causing it to fall off. Either treatment causes slight pain. But the result will be smoother skin and a more youthful appearance.

Q. *How should I treat spider veins on my legs?*
A. The thin, spidery bluish red or red veins that often appear on the thighs, knees, or feet are simply enlarged veins. These blood vessels (which are smaller than the larger blue varicose veins) become engorged and visible often because of pressure from standing, leg crossing, or excess weight. Pregnancy and hormonal treatments (birth control pills and hormone replacement therapy) can also contribute to spider veins because of the increase in estrogen in the body. If your mom had spider veins, you're likely to get them, too.

There are two ways to treat spider veins: injections (sclerotherapy) or laser therapy. With sclerotherapy, a dermatologist injects a solution that makes the veins clot, collapse, and dissolve. Depending on the severity of your problem, you may need repeat injections over a number of weeks. If the veins are particularly small, laser therapy can be effective. But this treatment is less desirable because it is more likely to cause bruising or discoloration. Support stockings and camouflaging leg makeup can also help.

Q. *What causes dark circles under my eyes and what can I do about them?*
A. Nothing makes a woman look more tired than dark under-eye circles. But a lack of sleep isn't the only cause. These darkened circles may be hereditary. The most common cause is probably the poor drainage of blood from the eye area. The good news is you can take several steps to reduce or camouflage them:

- First, try camouflaging dark circles by patting a concealer that is a shade lighter than your foundation on the under-eye area. Set the concealer with a loose powder.
- If circles are prominent, apply an eye cream containing moisturizers, alphahydroxy acids, and/or vitamin A to exfoliate and tighten under-eye skin. Ones to try are L'Oreal Hydra Fresh Circle Eraser and Clinique Anti-Gravity Firming Eye Lift.
- As a last resort, try to lighten the darkened skin with a bleaching agent such as hydroquinone. Ask your dermatologist for a recommendation. The bleaching agent should be applied twice a day for three months. Caution: Be very careful not to get the product in your eyes. Severe, persistent dark circles can also be treated with facial peels (glycolic acid, amino fruit acid, microdermabrasion); consult a dermatologist.

To reduce under-eye puffiness, be sure to get sufficient rest and try applying cool compresses (cucumber slices or damp lemon or chamomile tea bags) for several minutes before putting on makeup. Puffiness may be due to pads of fat beneath the eyes. In that case, surgical removal of the fat can help. If you have allergies that contribute to puffiness and redness, take your medication regularly.

Q. *Can I get rid of a mole safely and without leaving a scar?*
A. If you don't like the appearance or location of a mole, you can have it removed safely. Depending on the type of mole, its size, and its location, a dermatologist or plastic surgeon can shave the mole off or cut and stitch it. This process takes only a few minutes in the doctor's office. Mole removal is a quick way to make your skin look more clear and smooth. But the risks of discoloration and scarring must be considered. Don't have a mole removed if you have ever formed a keloidal scar.

Q. *Is there any way to prevent or treat stretch marks?*
A. Stretch marks are not harmful to the skin but they can be unsightly. The marks are caused by the excessive stretching of the skin that occurs during pregnancy, sig-

nificant weight loss or weight gain, or during growth spurts. They can be particularly noticeable—and distressing—for women of color because of the contrast between our natural skin tone and the typically lighter stretch marks.

You can't prevent or completely remove stretch marks, but you can try to minimize their appearance. Treatments work best when stretch marks are relatively new. The most effective treatment is the pulsed-dye laser, a procedure in which a laser beam is used to stimulate the production of collagen and elastin, proteins in the skin that are responsible for maintaining elasticity. These new proteins replace the damaged ones. Bruising can occur after treatment but will fade in a matter of days or weeks. The primary concern with skin of color is the possibility of discoloration. Topical treatments such as Retin-A or alphahydroxy acids may also help minimize the marks.

Case in Point: Growths Be Gone!

Joan came to my office concerned about little brown growths that stuck out from her neck, catching on her necklaces and shirt collars. The fifty-year-old Black woman also had developed flat growths on her cheeks that she felt were "taking over her face." Her mother had had similar growths. Joan wanted to have the growths removed, but she was afraid of the potential for pain and scarring. She'd also been told that removing the "skin tags" could cause her to bleed to death!

After I assured Joan that she would not bleed to death, we discussed the risk of scarring. Since she had no history of keloid formation and previous surgical scars had healed well, we decided to proceed. During two visits, I removed the growths from her neck and face with a surgical-grade scissor. Joan experienced some discomfort from the procedure but no pain. The growth areas healed in one week. The next time I saw her in my office Joan admitted that the removal of her skin tags was the best investment she'd ever made in herself. "They were ugly, uncomfortable, and annoying," she said. "I can't believe I waited so long to have them removed. I look ten years younger."

WINNING AGAINST WRINKLES

Though women of color can stave off those fine lines and deep wrinkles longer than White women can, we are not immune. Because of sun exposure and years of facial expressions, many Black women—especially those of us with lighter skin tones—will develop wrinkles. If these facial lines are troubling to you, and facial peels or microdermabrasion does not minimize them, you might consider anti-wrinkle treatments such as Botox or collagen injections. These techniques are less extensive than face-lifts and carry fewer risks. The treatment you select depends on the location of the wrinkles. Injections should be administered by an experienced dermatologist.

Forehead Wrinkles and Crow's-feet. The best treatment for wrinkles in the upper third of the face is Botox. In this procedure, a dermatologist injects a neurotoxin called botulinum (hence the name Botox) into the muscles beneath the wrinkled area. The toxin works by disrupting the signal from the nerves that normally tell facial muscles to contract. When you smile or make other facial expressions after a Botox treatment, the facial muscles remain relaxed and the skin does not wrinkle. A Botox injection takes only a few seconds and can last from three to six months. A temporary drooping of the eyelids is a possible but infrequent side effect, as is bruising. The fee for this procedure depends on the number of facial areas treated, but one area will cost between $350 and $450.

Laugh Lines, Lip Lines. The wrinkles in this area of the face—which are caused by skin thinning and gravity as opposed to muscle movement—can be treated by filler substances. The most commonly used filler substance is usually taken from collagen in cows or humans. A dermatologist will inject the substance in the dermis, or middle layer of the skin, in order to fill in or plump up facial lines and depressions. The collagen is later absorbed into the body. The treatment does not take long and lasts for three to six months. Some patients develop allergic reactions (bumps, redness) to bovine collagen; in those cases, human collagen can be used. The cost of collagen injections is similar to Botox, about $400.

Women over the age of thirty-five, whose skin is thinner than younger women, may benefit from another filler substance—fat. A treatment known as autologous fat transfer works by using the patient's own body fat to fill in deep lines. After injecting anesthesia, the doctor uses a syringe to extract fat from the abdomen, hip, or buttocks. Then the fat is injected into the wrinkled areas in the lower half of the face, filling in lines and wrinkles. (Fat transfers can also be used on other parts of the body such as the backs of hands.) Some of the extracted fat can be stored for later use. Autologous fat transfer treatments take longer than collagen injections, but since the fat is bulkier than collagen, the effects tend to last longer—from six months to a few years. Bruising and swelling may occur. The cost is between $1,000 and $1,500.

SKIN SOLUTIONS CHART

This simple chart provides at-a-glance answers to some common skin problems.

PROBLEM	SOLUTIONS	RISKS	RECOVERY TIME	COST
Dark spots (hyperpigmentation)	AHA/BHA creams	Dryness/irritation	None	$30 for 1 oz.
	AHA/BHA peels	Irritation/redness	None	$550–$700
	Microdermabrasion	Hyperpigmentation	None	$150 or more
	Laser resurfacing	Infection, scarring, hyperpigmentation	1–2 weeks	$2,000–$2,400
Blackheads/ clogged pores	AHA/BHA creams	Dryness/irritation	None	$30 for 1 oz.
	AHA/BHA peels	Irritation/redness	None	$550–$700
	Microdermabrasion	Hyperpigmentation	None	$150 or more
Acne scars/ chicken pox scars	Dermabrasion	Hyperpigmentation	None	$1,000–$1,500
	Laser resurfacing	Infection, scarring, hyperpigmentation	1–2 weeks	$2,000–$2,400

Fine lines, wrinkles	AHA/BHA peels	Irritation/redness	None	$550–$700
	Microdermabrasion	Hyperpigmentation	None	$150 or more
	Laser resurfacing	Infection, scarring, hyperpigmentation	1–2 weeks	$2,000–$2,400
	Botox or collagen injection	Drooping eyelids	None	$350–$450
	Fat injections	Bruising, swelling	None	$1,000–$1,500
Stretch marks	Retin-A	Irritation, dryness	None	$76 for 45g*
	AHA cream	Irritation with overuse	None	$30 for 1 oz.**
	Laser therapy	Bruising, scarring, hyperpigmentation	1–2 weeks	approx. $395
Spider veins	Sclerotherapy	Scarring, discoloration	None	$225–$250
	Laser therapy	Bruising, scarring, hyperpigmentation	1–2 weeks	$427***

Range of costs are according to the American Society of Dermatologic Surgery.

*Estimated average wholesale price of Retin-A, according to *American Family Physician*.

**Estimated average cost, according to American Academy of Cosmetic Surgery.

***Estimated average cost, according to American Society for Aesthetic Plastic Surgery.

COSMETIC SURGERY

If you still have appearance concerns that skin-care products or noninvasive procedures have not resolved, you may want to consider cosmetic surgery. If you feel cosmetic surgery will improve your looks and make you feel better about yourself, I encourage to look into it. Once thought of as luxuries reserved for models and millionaires, cosmetic surgical techniques have become more acceptable and affordable options for anyone who wants to look her best. From liposuction to breast implants, cosmetic procedures can target just about any area of the body, and in many cases they bring about positive improvements to many common appearance problems.

However, as women of color we must keep in mind that any injury or trauma to our skin can potentially trigger excess production of melanin and discoloration of the affected skin. That's why it's important to find a dermatologist or cosmetic surgeon who has experience treating skin of color. If you are prone to developing dark spots, be sure to discuss this with the physician you choose. You may need to use the bleaching agent hydroquinone should any discoloration occur and apply sunscreen to prevent further pigmentation problems. If you have had keloid scars, you should not consider cosmetic surgery because of the risk of additional scarring. If, however, you still want the procedure, ask the doctor to begin a series of cortisone injections to the scar each month for six months beginning three weeks after the surgery.

Before you schedule a procedure, discuss all the potential risks with your dermatologist or cosmetic surgeon. Be sure the physician has credentials, such as board certification in plastic or cosmetic surgery, and extensive experience (see "Questions to Ask the Doctor," page 114). Don't proceed until you are comfortable with the risk involved as well as the recovery time and cost. Here's a rundown of common procedures (the approximate costs listed here are based on surveys conducted by the American Academy of Cosmetic Surgery).

- *Liposuction*: A procedure in which a physician uses thin metal or plastic rods (cannulas) and a machine to suction excess fat from the neck, chest, back, arms, abdomen, thighs, buttocks, hips, knees, or calves/ankles of a patient. Risks: bleeding, infection, skin discoloration, numbness, scarring, uneven skin surface. Recovery time: several weeks. Average cost: $4,000.
- *Nose surgery* (rhinoplasty): By making small incisions in the nose, a physician manipulates bone and cartilage to reduce nose size or alter its shape or angle. Local or general anesthesia. Risks: swelling, bruising. Recovery time: several weeks. Cost: $4,000.
- *Eye, brow, and forehead lift* (blepharoplasty): A physician removes excess fat from sagging eyelids and folds under and around the eyes. Excess skin is removed from creased brows and forehead before they are "lifted." Risk: swelling, bruising.

Recovery time: a week to ten days; full benefit may not be seen for months. Cost: $3,000 for eyelids alone; $3,000 for forehead.

- *Face-lift* (rhytidectomy): After making incisions along the hairline and around the ears, a physician "lifts" sagging facial tissue and skin, then closes incisions. Risks: swelling, discoloration, numbness. Recovery time: several weeks. Cost: $5,000.

- *Breast augmentation* (augmentation mammaplasty): After making an incision under the breast or near the armpit, a physician lifts breast tissue and inserts an implant (usually a silicone shell filled with saline). Risks: pain, infection, swelling, skin discoloration, scarring. Breast implants can also rupture or deflate, and they do not last a lifetime. Recovery time: several weeks. Cost: $4,500.

- *Breast reduction* (reduction mammaplasty): A physician makes incisions around the breast in order to remove excess fat and skin and improve contour of breasts. Risks: swelling, discoloration, scarring, inability to nurse. Recovery time: several weeks. Cost: $5,000.

- *Tummy tuck* (abdominoplasty): A physician makes incisions along the abdomen in order to tighten loose muscles and remove excess fat and skin. Risks: bleeding, infection, reaction to anesthesia, tissue loss and fluid buildup under skin. Recovery time: several weeks. Cost: $5,000.

CHAPTER 6

LOOKING OUR BEST FROM THE INSIDE OUT

Your desire to look your best—youthful, radiant, confident—is enhanced by good health habits. The way you eat, exercise your body, and cope with stress has a direct impact on the health of your skin, hair, and nails. In fact, the first signs of illness often manifest on the skin. For that reason, along with your programs for skin, hair, and nails, you'll need to follow a balanced lifestyle regimen. But don't worry: you won't necessarily need to make radical, time-consuming changes. Just a few adjustments may make the difference and give you clearer skin and stronger, more lustrous hair and nails.

Despite our advances in education and in the workplace, many Black women suffer from diminished health. African-American women have higher rates of many illnesses, including ones that can affect the skin, such as obesity, diabetes, and lupus. We also often take medications that can impact skin health. As mothers and career women, we face high levels of stress. But whatever your current health status, most of our health challenges can be either prevented or at least managed with healthy lifestyle practices, including a sound diet, regular physical activity, and stress-reducing practices. What's good for our inner selves—our bodies and spirits—will benefit our outer appearance as well.

To evaluate your habits and bring into focus adjustments you may need to make, take this quick lifestyle quiz.

Quiz: *What Is Your Lifestyle?*

Answer yes or no to the following questions.

1. Do you drink several (seven-eight) glasses of plain water per day?
2. Do you get some form of exercise three or more days a week?
3. Do you take a daily multivitamin/mineral supplement?
4. Do you sleep approximately eight hours on most nights?
5. Do you take steps to reduce stress (take breaks, breathe deeply, meditate) every day or on most days?
6. Do you avoid or limit intake of caffeinated coffee, tea, or soda to no more than two cups (or two eight-ounce cans) per day?
7. Do you avoid or limit alcohol (wine, mixed drink, beer) to no more than two to three drinks per week?
8. Do you abstain from cigarettes and avoid secondhand smoke?
9. Do you eat several servings (at least five) of vegetables or fruit each day? (A serving usually fits in the palm of your hand.)
10. Do you feel good about yourself and optimistic about your life?

Answers

If you said yes to most of the questions, your lifestyle is looking great. If, however, you said yes to fewer than half, you're probably like most busy, stressed-out women. Your health and your skin will benefit from making a few small changes, such as carrying a water bottle wherever you go, adopting a midday walking routine, or going to bed a half hour earlier each night. This chapter describes additional strategies for improving your well-being.

NUTRITIONAL NEEDS

What does a healthy eating plan look like? It's balanced and comprises foods that offer a variety of nutrients your body needs to function well, supply you with energy, and keep you strong and free from illness. Those foods include, of course, the major nutrients—carbohydrates, proteins, and fats. The other essential nutrient we often forget is water. Here's a breakdown of what you should eat every day based on the U.S.D.A.'s Food Guide Pyramid:

- *Grains* (six to eleven servings) Whole-grain cereals, brown rice, oatmeal, barley, whole-grain breads, pastas, and crackers.
- *Vegetables* (three to five servings) Leafy salad greens, broccoli, spinach, carrots, peppers, asparagus, eggplant, potatoes, squash, snap peas, yams, corn.
- *Fruit* (two to four servings) Apples, oranges, pears, strawberries, melons, bananas, kiwi, grapefruit, berries, papaya, plums, nectarines, dried fruit.
- *Protein* (two to three servings) Fish, shellfish, chicken, turkey, beef, soybeans, peas.
- *Dairy* (two to three servings) Low-fat milk, cheese, yogurt.
- *Fats* (sparingly) Oils, butter.

What Did You Eat Today?

Many of us think our diet is basically healthy until we take a good look at it—or we notice a few extra pounds. Do a quick check. Write down what you ate today (or yesterday if today is unusual). Compare it to the Food Guide Pyramid recommendations. Are you getting enough protein? Too much fat? The right amount of veggies? If not, take note of it and tomorrow make up for what you missed.

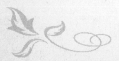

Water: The Good Skin Nutrient

H_2O is an essential nutrient, which means your body requires it every day to function at its best. Water aids in just about every bodily function, including digestion, circulation, temperature control, and elimination, among others. Because your body does not immediately signal thirst, and because you're probably used to ignoring the signal, you may be chronically dehydrated and not even know it. But dehydration will make you fatigued and even prone to illness.

If you are dehydrated, your skin will tend to look dull and lifeless. It might even have a gray or bluish cast. Your nails can also become dehydrated, turning brittle and weak. This dehydration may be caused by factors we don't often think of: drinking too much caffeinated coffee, tea, or soda; taking water pills for hypertension; exercising or simply walking around a lot on a hot day.

How can water benefit your skin? It hydrates skin cells, the building blocks of your skin. If you have dry skin, drinking lots of water—in addition to using moisturizer—will combat an ashen appearance. Hydration also keeps skin cells looking plump, minimizing the appearance of those fine lines on the forehead or around the eyes and mouth.

To get in the habit of drinking enough water,

- Keep a tall glass by your bed to remind yourself to drink up first thing in the morning and at night. By the end of the day, you should have had six to eight glasses.
- Carry bottled water in your purse or bag.
- Drink water with each meal. That's three glasses right there.
- Substitute water for caffeinated soda and coffee. Caffeine dehydrates the skin.
- Invest in a water-purifying pitcher or equipment for the freshest taste.
- Drink water flavored with lemon or lime, seltzer water, or herbal tea for variety.

Supplements: The Ultimate "Health Insurance"

While vitamin and mineral supplements are not substitutes for the healthy, balanced diet I described earlier, they can help fill in the gaps when you don't eat well or don't eat enough to satisfy your nutrient needs. Studies show that many Americans don't get adequate amounts of vital nutrients. And women have special nutritional needs, such as for calcium, iron, and folic acid. Certain antioxidant vitamins, including vitamins A, C, and E, are critical for health and benefit the skin by combating cell-damaging free radicals.

The best way to supplement is to take a multivitamin/mineral supplement daily. Shop for formulas designed for women and follow the instructions for dosage. If you're interested in taking additional supplements, discuss it first with your health-care provider or a nutritionist to make sure you really need extra supplementation and to avoid any negative interactions with medications you take. In certain cases, I've recommended vitamins for patients with acne or vitiligo. If you have either condition, discuss supplementation with your physician. But you must be careful not to take too much of certain vitamins, such as vitamin A, or side effects could develop.

EXERCISING YOUR OPTIONS

Too few women of color get the amount of physical activity we all need to be fit, feel energetic, and prevent illness. Having a super-busy schedule is one reason, but there are others—lack of motivation, self-consciousness, limited access to facilities, or worries about what sweating will do to your hair (see "Sweat and Our Hair," page 130). But exercise is not something we can avoid for long without consequences, such as weight gain, low energy, and poor sleep, among others. Women who don't exercise are at higher risk for nearly every major disease, including those that plague Black women at higher rates than White women: heart disease, diabetes, hypertension, and stroke.

Regular physical activity is also good for your skin, hair, and nails because, for one, it increases circulation, which brings oxygen and vital nutrients to your cells. Exercise improves sleep, which may minimize those under-eye circles. It's also been proven to help lower anxiety and stave off bouts of the blues or depression. When you feel better, you look better.

If you don't now get twenty to thirty minutes of physical activity every other day (three to four days each week), here's my advice for fitting fitness into your life. (If you have not exercised in years or have a chronic condition, talk to your physician first.):

1. Walk all day. Walk reasonable distances instead of driving or taking public transportation. Get off the bus or subway a stop or two early. Take the stairs in public places instead of escalators or elevators. Whenever you have the option to walk, do so.

2. Schedule your exercise routine like an appointment. Write it into your day planner and stick to it. If you can't work out one day during the week, make up for lost time the next day or on weekends.

3. Exercise in the morning to get it done and out of the way. Get up a half hour earlier to make time for it before dealing with breakfast, the kids, etc.

4. Work out in short spurts. If you can't spare a half hour, divide the time into two fifteen-minute workouts. Try a quick exercise video in the morning before work, then power walk during your lunch hour or after work.

5. Get equipped. Invest in home exercise equipment—a treadmill, stair climber, or stationary bike, for example. This way you can sneak in twenty minutes or more without having to leave home. Buy some light free weights while you're at it.

6. Enlist the family. Spend time with your mate and kids by working out together. On weekends, go for a hike, roller blade or ice skate, or play a sport (touch football, softball, basketball) as a family.

7. Get moving! In your spare time, lift free weights, do lunges, or simply touch your toes to get a good stretch. It's all exercise.

Sweat and Our Hair

Like many women of color, you may avoid vigorous exercise because of the havoc sweat wreaks on your hair. But physical activity is essential to your well-being—and the health of your skin, hair, and nails. Before a workout; wash your face with a gentle cleanser for your skin type to remove makeup that could clog pores. To keep your hair looking good, pull it back loosely—not too tight—to reduce the amount of oils that come in contact with your face. Always carry a white cotton towel during workouts to blot perspiration. After your workout, shower quickly and moisturize your skin as needed.

Once you've established a three-day-a-week routine for cardiovascular exercise, add resistance training and stretching to make your workout complete. Keep it fun and challenging by trying different forms of exercise and by periodically increasing the difficulty or duration of your regimen. Here are some old and new ideas for ways to work it out:

- *Cardiovascular workout* (twenty to thirty minutes, three to five days a week): Power walking on a treadmill or outdoors; jogging; cycling or spinning; aerobics; salsa, jazz, funk, or African dance classes; jumping rope; kickboxing; exercise tapes.
- *Resistance training* (twenty to thirty minutes, at least two days a week): Free weights; exercise machines; calisthenics; resistance bands; body bars; medicine balls.
- *Flexibility and balance* (at least as often as you do cardio and resistance, or every day): Basic stretching; yoga; tai chi; qigong; exercise balls.

Weighing In on Weight Issues

Research shows that the majority of African-American women are overweight and a disproportionate number of us are obese. This excess weight contributes to the high rates of serious medical problems (diabetes, heart disease, stroke) among Black women and puts otherwise healthy women at risk. Being heavy can also diminish our energy; contribute to knee, ankle, and foot pain; and make it harder to perform other activities of daily living such as climbing stairs.

In terms of our appearance, excess weight stretches the skin. As the skin's elastin fibers break, stretch marks appear. Though not harmful, stretch marks are difficult to treat and impossible to completely remove. When significant weight is lost, our skin does not automatically snap back. The excess skin not only may have stretch marks but also may sag and in some cases require surgical removal.

If you're overweight or you're not sure, visit your physician to discuss it and to make sure there is no underlying condition contributing to your weight gain. Together, you can determine a healthy weight for your age, height, and body frame, and set goals for weight loss if necessary. Most experts recommend losing no more than two pounds per week. The safest way to shed pounds and keep them off for good is to increase physical activity (see "Exercising Your Options," page 128) and decrease excess fat and calories in your diet. Keep an eye on your portions to make sure you don't overeat. Small changes in your habits will help: eat one roll instead of two or a half a pat of butter on bread instead of one or two pats.

A GOOD NIGHT'S SLEEP

As busy women, we tend to take sleep for granted and turn to stimulants (coffee, diet soda) to get us going when we're tired. But most people need a solid eight hours a night in order to wake refreshed and to perform at their best. Lack of sleep makes us less alert during the day, and it interferes with our ability to concentrate and be productive. It can make us careless, resulting in preventable accidents. A sleepy person also is often an irritable person who does not get along as well with her family, friends, or colleagues. In the face of life's demands, the body perceives sleep deprivation as "stress." Sufficient, sound sleep is important for our health and overall quality of life.

Sleep is also a natural and free beauty aid. When we're tired, our eyes can become red and puffy. Dark under-eye circles can form or become more pronounced.

Our skin may look more pale and lifeless. If you are chronically sleep-deprived, no amount of makeup will hide it. But a good night's sleep will help you wake up renewed.

If you have ongoing problems with sleep, such as insomnia, sleep apnea (breathing difficulties during sleep), or restless leg syndrome, see your doctor for treatment. Sleep can also be diminished if you suffer from major stress, heartburn, depression, or other disorders, so get a checkup to make sure your health problems are addressed. Otherwise, you may need to simply make sleep more of a priority. Follow these tips for a good night's rest:

- Avoid drinking caffeine and alcohol in the evening. The caffeine may prevent you from falling asleep and alcohol may cause you to wake up prematurely.
- Don't eat a big meal right before bedtime. If you are hungry, try a light carbohydrate snack. Avoid chocolate, which contains caffeine.
- Stop smoking. Smokers have more difficulty falling asleep and experience nicotine withdrawal during the night.
- Exercise. Physical activity can deepen sleep. Just don't do it two to three hours before bedtime.
- Relax before bedtime. Take a warm bath or read a good book. Turn off the TV; watching television may keep you up later than your body really wants to be.
- Stick to a routine. Try waking and going to bed at the same times to maintain regular sleep patterns.

STRESS IN CHECK

Emotional stress is an ever-present part of women's lives. Work pressure, family responsibilities, financial strain, and relationship difficulties all contribute to making us feel stressed out. When we're under pressure, our bodies release stress-related hormones to help us respond and cope. However, when we experience too much stress and no relief, our immune systems start to break down. The stress overload can contribute to a host of physical and emotional health problems, from frequent headaches and colds to more serious conditions such as hypertension.

Excessive amounts of stress can also be hard on your skin and hair. The flux of stress hormones may trigger mild to severe acne outbreaks or hives. Ongoing stress can also cause unsightly cold sores to develop on the lips. If stress becomes severe, two types of hair loss—telogen effluvium and alopecia areata—can occur.

The sources of the stress in your life may not be easy to change, but you can change the way you cope. Instead of letting stress get to you, learn how to manage it.

Stress Stoppers

- Breathe deeply. For ten to thirty minutes a day, find a quiet space at home or work and pay attention to your breathing. Close your eyes and count to 10 as you slowly breathe in and out.
- Sip a calming herbal tea. A warm mug of chamomile or valerian tea with honey will help relax you.
- Keep a journal. Putting your thoughts on paper is an easy, effective form of emotional release. Invest in a decorative journal book and pen; write once a day.
- Call a good friend. During a stressful period, don't forget to call on those friends who make you laugh and help you see the lighter side of life.
- Get a pet. Focusing your thoughts and energies on a furry animal can take your mind off stressful events.
- Join a support group. Seek out a group with similar concerns or interests, such as a book club, knitting network, or twelve-step group.
- Meditate. Gaze at a candle, repeat a mantra (Ohm), or simply empty your mind for ten to thirty minutes for instant relaxation.
- Say a little prayer. Don't wait until Sunday to hand your concerns over to your God or a Higher Power through prayer.
- Do something silly. Instead of fretting over a problem, distract yourself with your favorite comic strip, humor book, or a funny movie rental.

- Say no to the negative. Keep your distance from those friends and family members who always see the glass half-empty. Negative thinking is contagious.

- Join a spiritual community. A local church, mosque, or other house of worship may offer a supportive community and new friendships, as well as spiritual reinforcement.

- Carve out time for yourself. Take twenty minutes for a bubble bath at night or for a solitary stroll at the end of the day. Better yet, schedule a monthly massage.

- Take a walk in nature. A visit to the local park or beach may make you feel instantly calmer.

- Get counseling. When stress is simply overwhelming and interfering with your enjoyment of life, seek the care of a mental-health care provider.

A GORGEOUS ATTITUDE

We often hear that beauty comes from within. The efforts you make to take good care of yourself physically and emotionally will help your natural beauty shine through. As you put your beauty and self-care programs into practice, you'll begin to look better and feel more self-assured. But if you still don't feel positive about your appearance, you may need to examine and challenge some deeply ingrained beliefs. Instead of succumbing to thoughts like "I wish I had a smaller/bigger nose" or "I hate my hair," keep in mind that your self-image is at least in part influenced by artificial media images—images that don't reflect the full range of *our* natural beauty.

Focus on those aspects of yourself that you like. If friends always compliment your great smile or lovely nails, take pride in those assets. As your self-image improves, you can work on accepting your skin, hair, and body the way they are. Having a positive attitude about your appearance and your life will go a long way toward making your natural radiance and beauty apparent for all to see.

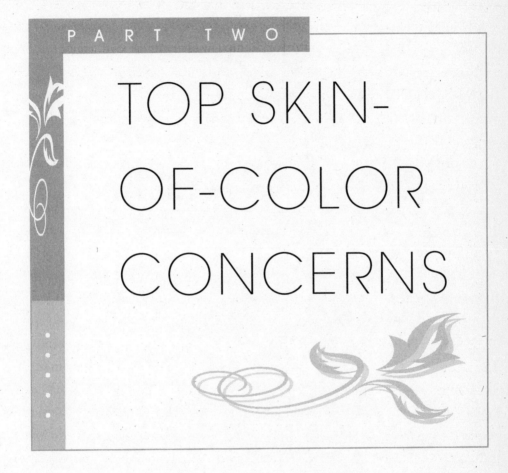

PART TWO

TOP SKIN-OF-COLOR CONCERNS

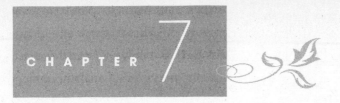

CHAPTER 7

SKIN 911

Your skin of color is remarkably resilient and protective, yet it's more susceptible to being damaged by common skin problems. With brown skin, a number of everyday skin conditions and diseases can stimulate our production of melanin and lead to the development of disfiguring dark spots. These discolorations may be difficult to treat and harmful to our appearance and our self-esteem.

In skin of color, some very common conditions have a distinctly different appearance as compared to white skin, and they can be hard to detect. A disease that causes redness in white skin may make skin of color darker or lighter. The symptoms of illness may also differ in terms of location on the body, size, and texture. These dissimilarities can mask problems and lead to delayed diagnosis or even misdiagnosis. Because the signs of many serious diseases first develop on the skin, recognizing signs of illness on your skin is critical to your health.

Even if you have a relatively healthy, blemish-free complexion, you've probably been plagued by at least one of the conditions described in this chapter. The key to keeping your skin of color clear and radiant is to pay attention to signs of change in your skin, seek treatment at the drugstore or doctor's office, and take steps to prevent problems in the future. By actively monitoring and protecting your skin, you'll minimize the risk of discolorations and scars that can be hard to get rid of. You'll also have the confidence that comes from knowing that you look your absolute best.

SKIN, HAIR, AND NAIL PROBLEMS AND THEIR SOLUTIONS

Allergic Reactions

- *Symptoms:* Red, itchy skin. An allergic reaction may take the form of small brown bumps, larger red bumps, or raised welts known as hives, and last for several minutes to several days.
- *Causes:* Allergies to medications, food, insect bites, dyes; exposure to skin-care products or cosmetics; exposure to poison ivy or poison oak.
- *Treatment:* Cool compresses. Over-the-counter calamine lotion, corticosteroids, and antihistamines such as Benadryl. See your doctor if a rash does not subside or improve within a few days, becomes encrusted or weepy, or if the allergic reaction is severe enough to affect your breathing or swallowing.
- *Prevention:* Avoidance of allergy causes listed above.

Cold Sores or Fever Blisters (Herpes Simplex)

- *Symptoms:* Red, raised fluid-filled blisters that typically appear on the lips. Blisters are usually preceded by tingling, discomfort, or pain in the area. Cold sores typically last seven to ten days as blisters grow, break, crust, and slough off. Cold sores can also develop on the nose, cheeks, or fingers, or inside the mouth.
- *Causes:* Herpes simplex virus type 1, a common virus. (herpes simplex virus type 2 usually causes genital herpes.) The virus is highly contagious and spreads through contact with an infected individual or a fomite (infected inanimate object). Once you catch the virus, it will lie dormant in your body. Under certain circumstances such as stress, illness (especially associated with fever), and sunlight, it will reactivate and come to the surface.
- *Treatment:* Cold sores usually clear up on their own within a week, but the virus is not curable and can cause future sores. Prescription antiviral ointments or pills

can help speed the healing of frequently recurring sores. Over-the-counter painkillers or ice might also relieve discomfort. You may find drugstore products such as Blistex or Campho-Phenique soothing to your irritated and inflamed lips.

- *Prevention:* Avoid kissing or close contact with others while blisters are forming, present, or healing. Wash your hands frequently and avoid touching your mouth and then touching other parts of your body. Don't pick at blisters. Use a lip balm with sunblock on your lips year-round.

Foot Odor

- *Symptoms:* Pungent, persistent odor emanating from feet.
- *Causes:* Sweating; growth of bacteria or fungi on feet, especially feet trapped in tight shoes.
- *Treatment:* If odor is accompanied by other symptoms such as itching, burning, blisters, or discolored nails, see your doctor. You may have athlete's foot or a bacterial or fungal infection that requires medication.
- *Prevention:* Wash feet, including between toes, with antibacterial soap. Dry feet and sprinkle antifungal foot powder on feet and in shoes. Don only cotton socks; change your socks during the day if you sweat a lot, and remove pantyhose as soon as your workday ends. Discard old smelly shoes.

Genital Warts *(Condyloma accuminatum)*

- *Symptoms:* Skin-colored or pink growths that develop in the genital area, including the vulva, vagina, cervix, or anus. Warts can grow in clusters resembling cauliflower or broccoli. They are contagious and spread through sexual contact as well as from mother to child during delivery. Genital warts may also develop in the mouth or throat after oral sex.
- *Causes:* A virus known as human papilloma virus, or HPV. Without treatment, HPV can lead to abnormal cell changes in the cervix that are detected through

an abnormal pap smear. Genital warts can lead to cervical cancer in some cases so they must be treated.

- **Treatment:** Your physician may use either topical medications or surgery to remove warts, depending on their location and size. Surgical options include laser surgery, cryotherapy (freezing with liquid nitrogen), or electrocautery (electrical burning). The application of topical medications such as Aldara, Condolox, or Podophyllin is a painless alternative. If your partner has been infected, it is imperative that he or she be treated as well.
- **Prevention:** Avoid spreading warts by refraining from sexual activity while warts are visible. Never engage in unprotected sexual intercourse: condom use is a must for the prevention of genital warts. Prompt diagnosis and treatment of genital warts is one of several reasons it's important for women of color to get regular gynecological exams, including Pap smears. Look for the release of a new vaccine for HPV.

Ingrown Toenails

- **Symptoms:** Pain or tenderness in the toe (most often the big toe). Redness or pus may develop if infection develops.
- **Causes:** Curved nails, tight shoes, improper nail trimming.
- **Treatment:** Over-the-counter ingrown toenail treatments; antibiotic ointment; saltwater foot soaks to reduce inflammation. In severe cases, your doctor may need to remove the ingrown portion of the nail and prescribe oral antibiotics.
- **Prevention:** Trim toenails straight across. Avoid wearing tight shoes or socks.

Nail Fungus

- **Symptoms:** Initially a fungal infection begins with a tiny white or yellow spot on the nail. The nail will eventually become thickened with debris or material beneath the nail's surface. It may turn yellow, green, brown, or black and become crumbly. Nails often separate from the underlying nail bed, giving a white appearance to the nail. Fungal infections are most common in toenails but also affect fingernails. Fingernail fungus is very common, especially in women who wear acrylic nails. ***Warning: A single black streak on one nail may indicate skin cancer in Hispanics and African Americans—see your doctor immediately.***

- ***Causes:*** A fungus infects the nail, using the nail keratin (protein cells that compose the nail) as fuel or food. Fungal infections are commonly spread in public facilities such as gyms, showers, and swimming pools.

- ***Treatment:*** Oral antifungal medications, which you will need to take for twelve weeks for toenail fungus or six weeks for fingernail infections. At the completion of therapy, the existing nails will not appear normal but as the new nail or nails grow, they will be normal. Although antifungal nail creams are not very effective for treating nail fungus, prescription antifungal nail lacquers may be helpful. The nail lacquers require daily use for six to twelve months.

- ***Prevention:*** Keep feet and toenails dry. Use antifungal powder regularly. Wear cotton socks and change them frequently if you sweat a lot. Avoid wearing damp socks or tight shoes in which fungi can grow. Protect your feet with waterproof footwear such as flip-flops or water shoes at public showers or swimming pools. For fingernail care, wash hands frequently and dry them thoroughly. Don't wear artificial nails for long periods of time, which may only mask and/or contribute to fungal infections. Only patronize nail salons with licensed practitioners and sanitized environments. Take your own nail implements with you each time you go to the manicurist.

Pityriasis Alba

- ***Symptoms:*** Round patches of lightened skin covered with fine scales. Pityriasis alba tends to appear on the face. It is most common in children and adolescents but also occurs in adulthood.

- ***Causes:*** Pityriasis alba is a form of mild eczema. Though discoloration is temporary, it can be distressing for people of color. Sun exposure may make it more noticeable.

- *Treatment:* Hydrocortisone or other steroid creams.
- *Prevention:* Good emollients or lotions may help to make pityriasis alba less apparent.

Scabies

- *Symptoms:* Intense itching that awakens you from sleep at night. Itchy bumps of various sizes or thin marks (called burrows) on skin. Scabies is most likely to appear on your extremities (wrists, finger web spaces) but can develop anywhere on the body, such as around the waist or on the nipples.
- *Causes:* A mite (tiny insect) that burrows under the skin. Scabies spreads from person to person or through contact with the infected person, their clothes or other personal items. Scabies tends to afflict sexual partners, entire families, or classrooms.
- *Treatment/prevention:* Prescription creams or lotions such as Elimite or Kwell. Wash all clothing and bedding that came into contact during the previous five days in hot water, then dry in high heat to kill mites. Treat all infected family members at the same time and repeat the treatment after seven days.

Seborrheic Dermatitis

- *Symptoms:* Red, light, or dark skin patches with scales and flakiness that appear on the scalp, hairline, behind the ears or in the ears, in the eyebrows, and along the sides of the nose. Seborrheic dermatitis can also develop on the chest.
- *Causes:* Excess oil, or sebum, in hair follicles. Yeast growth in sebum may also exacerbate the condition.
- *Treatment:* Seborrheic dermatitis is not curable but it can be managed. Medicated shampoos containing either ketoconazole, corticosteroids, salicylic acid, selenium sulfide, sulfur, coal tar, or other ingredients will help control scalp symptoms. Leave the shampoo on the scalp for several minutes before rinsing. Prescription corticosteroid creams, ointments, gels, solutions, oils, or foams are often used if shampoos are not effective alone.

- **Prevention:** You may need to alternate different medicated shampoos since they tend to lose their effectiveness over time.

Seborrheic Keratosis

- **Symptoms:** Brown growths that range in diameter from a pinhead to half-dollar. They often have a broccoli-like surface. The growths may develop in clusters on the cheeks, where they are called *dermatosis papulosa nigra*.
- **Causes:** The cause of keratoses is unknown but the growths tend to develop more commonly during pregnancy and as women mature. They often run in families, so heredity is a factor.
- **Treatment:** Seborrheic keratoses do not pose a threat to your health but they may be unsightly or uncomfortable. You should have growths examined by a physician to rule out skin cancer. They can then be removed through cryotherapy (freezing with liquid nitrogen), curettage (scraping), or electrosurgery (electrical burning) or minor surgical excision.
- **Prevention:** Since the cause is unknown, there is no way to prevent seborrheic keratoses.

Striae Distensae (stretch marks)

- **Symptoms:** Light-colored or red lines or marks that commonly appear during pregnancy but also develop after sudden weight gain or loss, and in adolescents during growth spurts. The marks most often appear on the lower abdomen, buttocks, thighs, shoulders, and on the sides of the breasts.
- **Causes:** Rapid stretching of skin, which damages the skin proteins collagen and elastin.
- **Treatment:** In general it's very difficult to eliminate stretch marks. Pulsed dye laser treatments that stimulate the production of new collagen and elastin may be used. Topical Retin-A, a vitamin A derivative, may also help minimize the appearance of stretch marks.

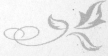

- **Prevention:** There is no way to prevent striae, but the sooner the marks are treated after they appear, the better the results.

Tinea Pedis (Athlete's Foot)

- **Symptoms:** A rash between the toes, on the soles, and on the sides of the feet characterized by flaking, peeling, or cracking of the skin. Blisters may develop. The area is very itchy and may burn. Often the toenails are discolored or ragged with fungal debris beneath the nails.
- **Causes:** Fungi that infect the superficial layer of skin. Athlete's foot fungi are commonly spread in public facilities such as gyms, showers, and swimming pools.
- **Treatment:** Topical antifungal cream, powder, or spray on infected areas. It's important to apply the cream to all areas of the foot, including between the toes. Oral antifungal medications may be necessary if the fungal infection is severe or if blisters have developed. Toenail fungus (*tinea ungium*) is most effectively treated with oral antifungal medication.
- **Prevention:** Keep feet dry. Use antifungal powder regularly, especially if athlete's foot is a recurring problem. Wear cotton socks and change them frequently if you sweat a lot. Avoid wearing damp socks or tight shoes in which fungi can grow. Protect your feet with waterproof footwear (flip-flops or water shoes) at public showers or swimming pools.

Tinea Versicolor

- **Symptoms:** White, red, or brown patches that develop most commonly on the trunk, neck, and extremities. Lesions may itch. Tinea versicolor may cause discoloration (hyperpigmentation or hypopigmentation) in brown skin and is usually worse in the summer.
- **Causes:** A type of yeast known as *Pityrosporum ovale*. This disease is most common in tropical, humid environments.

- *Treatment:* Topical medications including selenium sulfide and other antifungal creams, lotions, shampoos, or solutions. Persistent or recurring lesions may be treated with oral antifungal drugs.
- *Prevention:* Periodic use (once monthly) of antifungal products may also be beneficial in controlling yeast.

Torn Earlobes

- *Symptoms:* Tears in earlobe beginning where ears are pierced straight through the end of the lobe (or incomplete or partial tears).
- *Causes:* Heavy, dangling earrings that stretch the hole in lobes over time; yanked or pulled earrings.
- *Treatment:* Earlobe repair surgery or "reconstruction" done with sutures. A new ear hole can be created during the reconstruction or about three to six months after healing.
- *Prevention:* Wear lightweight pierced earrings or clip-on earrings.

Warts *(Verruca vulgaris)*

- *Symptoms:* Skin growths that appear most commonly on hands and feet, but can grow anywhere on the body and last months to years.
- *Causes:* A common virus, *human papilloma virus* (HPV), that spreads through person-to-person contact or contact with a surface where the virus is present.
- *Treatment:* Over-the-counter medications containing up to 20 percent salicylic acid. If salicylic acid does not work or if warts are particularly troublesome, they can be removed through surgery, laser surgery, cryotherapy (freezing with liquid nitrogen), or electrocautery (electrical burning), or via application of other topical medications recommended by your dermatologist.
- *Prevention:* Avoid spreading existing warts to other parts of the body by treating warts promptly and not using a razor on wart-infected skin. Do not pick,

pull, or bite the wart. If you use public showers at gyms or public swimming pools, protect your feet by wearing waterproof footwear.

SKIN SYMPTOMS THAT ARE MORE THAN SKIN DEEP

Your skin may be the first place signs of more serious illnesses appear. In many cases, such illnesses are more common among African Americans and Hispanics. Because symptoms are not always obvious, serious medical problems can go undetected and untreated for months or years. Here I describe diseases with symptoms that may manifest on your skin, hair, or nails.

Diabetes

If you have diabetes, your body lacks insulin or is unable to use the insulin that you have to process sugar for energy. Without treatment, diabetes can lead to several complications, including blindness, kidney failure, limb amputation, and death. Among the signs of diabetes are extreme thirst, frequent urination, and numbness or tingling in the feet or hands. Other symptoms include fatigue, blurred vision, dramatic weight loss, and recurrent yeast infections. There are several rashes associated with diabetes that can occur on the skin. With diabetic dermopathy, red and itchy patches can occur on the shins. Black velvety patches on the side and back of the neck, a condition known as acanthosis nigricans, can be an early sign of diabetes. If you have such symptoms, see your doctor immediately for diabetes screening. The American Diabetes Association estimates that nearly 11 percent of African Americans—or one in nine—have diabetes, and many of us don't know it.

Lupus

Women suffering from lupus (systemic lupus erythematosus or discoid lupus) have a difficult condition that causes the immune system to attack the body's organs and tissues instead of protecting them. Lupus afflicts Black and Native American women more than any other group for reasons that are not well understood. The disease can harm all organ systems of the body, including the skin, joints, kidneys, brain, lungs, and heart. Signs that develop on the skin include a butterfly-shaped rash across the face, pale or purple fingers and toes, sun sensitivity, and hair loss. Additional symptoms include malaise, joint pain, fever, chest pain, and nausea. One form of lupus, known as discoid lupus, primarily affects the skin. With discoid lupus, red, dark, or white atrophic (depressed) patches can form on the face, scalp, or ears. All forms of lupus may be difficult to diagnose and treat, so seek the care of a provider with experience treating the disease.

Sarcoidosis

Sarcoidosis is a disease that is characterized by the formation of abnormal collections of cells called *granulomas*. The granulomas can collect in the lungs, lymph nodes, liver, skin, and other organs and tissue. The symptoms of sarcoidosis can be mild or severe, depending on the individual. They include waxy brown bumps on the skin (especially the face), purplish patches on the nose, and extremely dry patches on the legs. Other symptoms include weakness, headaches, shortness of breath, painful joints, weight loss, swollen lymph nodes, chest pain, and sinus problems.

Sickle Cell Disease

Many people of color, but particularly African Americans, have the condition that is named after the sickle shape of some blood cells. These cells can clump together and impede circulation, causing severe pain and even death. Sickle cell disease can cause jaundice or a yellowing of the skin and the whites of the eyes; swelling in the feet and hands; leg sores or ulcers; stunted growth; painful joints; and severe pain in the chest, abdomen, arms, and legs.

Skin Cancer

Although skin cancer is far less common among Blacks and Hispanics than Whites, it can be just as deadly. In these groups, skin cancer may manifest as black bumps or spots on the extremities, including the palms, fingers, soles, and toes. While dark streaks on fingernails or toenails are normal for many Blacks and Hispanics, an ink-like streak or spot on a single nail could indicate cancer. The mouth and genitals are other areas where skin cancer might develop in individuals with skin of color. In addition to these signs, you should be on the lookout for moles or other growths that suddenly change in color, size, texture, or shape, and growths that ooze, bleed, or cause itching or pain.

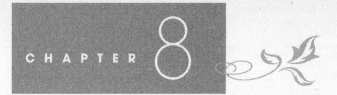

CHAPTER 8

PROBLEMS
WITH PIGMENT

Dark marks, blemishes, spots, patches, discolorations—
whatever you prefer to call them, these disorders of pigmentation have a damaging
psychological impact on women of color. While the natural pigmentation in your
skin provides several advantages—such as sun protection and fewer signs of aging—
it also has the disadvantage of being susceptible to developing devastating discolorations. Many common factors, including sunlight, injury, trauma, and even skin
disease, can either overstimulate or damage your pigment-producing skin cells.
When that occurs, those skin cells can produce too much or too little melanin and
discolorations appear. Dark or light spots develop in white skin as well, but these
discolorations are often not as dramatic as in people of color.

The most striking example of a disfiguring pigmentation problem is vitiligo,
a condition that causes milky-white patches of skin to emerge on the face or body.
In individuals with skin of color, the milky white patches are highly noticeable
against the brown or black skin. And there are other such disorders that have a
damaging psychological impact on women of color. But you'll be happy to know
that in many cases, these pigmentation problems can be treated successfully.

There are four pigmentation disorders that I commonly see in women of color:
postinflammatory hyperpigmentation (dark marks), postinflammatory hypopigmentation (light marks), melasma (the mask of pregnancy), and vitiligo. Learning about

the causes and treatments of these conditions will help you not only to prevent or manage skin discolorations but to cope with them as well. In this chapter, I'll discuss the impact of common cultural practices on skin discolorations. You'll also discover what doesn't work and the risks associated with some over-the-counter products. For example, certain skin bleaching agents, which are increasingly used by people of color in the United States and abroad, can cause serious side effects.

Case in Point: Extra-strength May Causa Extra Problems

As a woman of color, you'll need to be especially careful with the treatments you choose. Unfortunately, there are many women who come to me and report that a new product they were experimenting with burned their skin and caused dark marks. Carolyn was one such patient. At age thirty-five, in the midst of a divorce and while working overtime to make ends meet, she found that stress was causing her to break out in acne bumps on her cheeks. Despite having dry and sensitive skin, she used her seventeen-year-old son's extra-strength acne cleanser and his extra-strength topical acne medication. Her skin became inflamed with dryness, redness, and peeling as a result. When the inflammation subsided, she was left with large dark patches on her face—a problem known as postinflammatory hyperpigmentation. Before I began treatment to lighten her dark marks, I had Carolyn begin a regimen of Cetaphil cleanser and lotion twice daily for gentle cleansing. The type of hyperpigmentation she suffered could have been totally avoided if she had consulted a dermatologist, who would have selected the appropriate cleansing products and medications for her skin.

HYPERPIGMENTATION

Hyperpigmentation literally means "excessive pigmentation or darkening of the skin." Hyperpigmentation may develop all over the skin or in discrete patches.

In this condition, the melanocyte cells that normally produce brown pigment evenly across the skin go into overdrive, producing discoloration in spots, patches, or large areas of the skin. Hyperpigmentation may be triggered by a medical condition, certain medications, or external causes. For example, Minocin (minocycline), a commonly used oral antibiotic for the treatment of acne, can cause a bluish hyperpigmentation of the skin.

When the cause of the hyperpigmentation is irritation or inflammation of the skin, the condition is known as *postinflammatory hyperpigmentation*. The factors that cause postinflammatory hyperpigmentation are varied and include scratches, burns, rashes, pimples, acne, prescription as well as over-the-counter topical medications, various skin-care products, and surgery. Hyperpigmentation may also develop after cosmetic procedures such as chemical peels, laser hair removal, or a laser resurfacing procedure. Additionally, it can occur after the skin is irritated by skin-care products or cosmetics that are not designed for your skin type.

Once a dark mark or splotch develops, it may fade on its own. But as you have probably discovered, the natural fading process may take many months or even years. A survey we performed at the Skin of Color Center revealed that discolorations due to acne took an average of more than four months to fade without treatment.

Many women of color do not realize that repeated irritation, inflammation, or exposure to sunlight can make discolorations worsen or linger. That's why you should take the prevention of hyperpigmentation and the ongoing care of your skin seriously.

Possible Causes of Postinflammatory Hyperpigmentation

Injury (scratch, cut, burn, bruise)

Inflammation

Rash (eczema, pityriasis rosea, etc.)

Acne or pimples

Trauma

Surgery

Sunburn.

Hyperpigmentation may appear brown, black, gray, blue, or even blue–black in skin of color. If the pigmentation contrasts sharply with light to medium-toned skin, it can be particularly noticeable. The hue or color of the hyperpigmentation can indicate the location of the increased pigmentation within the skin—that is, in the upper portion of the skin, the epidermis, or in the deeper, dermal layer. Epidermal pigmentation tends to have a brownish hue; dermal pigmentation appears blue.

To determine the depth of the hyperpigmentation, your dermatologist can shine a special blue light (known as the Wood's light) on your skin. Identifying the level of the pigmentation is very important in terms of predicting treatment success. If the pigmentation is in the epidermal layer, there is effective treatment to remove the pigmentation. However, if the pigmentation is in the dermal layer, there is no effective treatment and it may take many years for the body to slowly remove the pigmentation naturally.

Case in Point: Undoing Discoloration

For a year, Michelle, age forty-two, had been suffering from hair growth and bumps under the chin. When she came to my office, she had just completed five laser hair removal treatments. As a result, she was experiencing minimal growth of chin hair and almost no bumps at all. Her primary concern was related to the dark marks where the bumps had been. These bumps were the result of postinflammatory hyperpigmentation. I examined her chin area with the Wood's light. The discoloration did appear darker under the Wood's light, indicating that the pigmentation was in the epidermal or upper skin layer. I explained that there were several effective medications that I could give her to lighten the hyperpigmentation. She began a course of Lustra Cream, which she applied morning and night. After three months the dark areas on Michelle's chin had faded nicely.

Myth: Dark marks can be scrubbed away.

Truth: Dark marks are the result of excessive melanin production—not dirt—
so they cannot be rubbed or scrubbed away. In fact, harsh scrubbing may
irritate skin of color, triggering the development of more dark marks. So stop
scrubbing your elbows and knees. That will not lighten them.

Treatment of Hyperpigmentation

If you've experienced hyperpigmentation that has not faded on its own, it's important to consult a dermatologist who can help you determine the cause of the discoloration, the location of the discoloration, and the best treatment for you. It's
essential that you understand that if your hyperpigmentation is caused by acne, for
example, you'll need to first treat the acne, then treat the dark marks. If you don't
treat the underlying problem, you will continue to develop new marks. Once the
underlying problem is treated or controlled, your doctor can select one of several
ways to lighten the dark skin spots or blotches and restore an even complexion to
your skin. Restoring an even skin tone is a process that may require several months
so you'll have to exercise patience and follow instructions.

Hydroquinone. One of the most effective ways to lighten dark marks or areas on
the skin is with a product containing hydroquinone, a chemical lightening agent.
These products come in 1 to 2 percent over-the-counter strengths and 3 to 4 percent prescription strengths. A dermatologist can recommend which strength to
use—usually one of the 4 percent hydroquinone products such as Lustra cream.
The hydroquinone cream, gel, or solution is applied carefully to the dark marks
only (avoiding the normal-appearing skin) once or twice a day. Treatment with hydroquinone should not extend beyond six months. (If the hydroquinone is going
to be effective, an improvement will be seen within six months.) Prolonged use of
hydroquinones can result in a paradoxical darkening of skin known as *exogenous
ochronosis*, a disfiguring condition that has no cure.

Some women are allergic to hydroquinone-containing products. To detect a possible allergic reaction, test the product on a small area of skin such as under the jawline or on the forearm. Follow the directions for patch-testing on the product label or follow your physician's instructions. Often patch-testing involves applying a small amount of the product to a limited area of the skin for several days. The development of redness, itching, or bumps up to seven days later indicates an allergic reaction and the product should not be used again.

To improve its efficacy, the hydroquinone may be combined with several other medications. These combinations may include:

Hydroquinone/sunscreen
Hydroquinone/kojic acid
Hydroquinone/glycolic acid
Hydroquinone/tretinoin/cortisone

The products containing these combinations are applied once or twice daily for several weeks of treatment.

Glycolic Acid. Whether in the form of a facial peel or in a cleanser, cream, lotion, gel, or solution, glycolic acid—an alphahydroxy acid (AHA)—works by gently exfoliating the uppermost layer of skin and dark marks along with it. You can find glycolic acid products, containing anywhere between 5 and 20 percent glycolic acid, in your drugstore or your dermatologist's office. Your dermatologist will be able to determine if glycolic acid is appropriate for your skin. If it is, you will be instructed to wash twice daily with the glycolic acid cleanser, followed by the glycolic cream, gel, lotion, or solution. You can expect to begin seeing results within four to eight weeks.

Again, patch-test the product on a small patch of skin to make sure that it does not cause irritation, redness, or a rash. Glycolic acid, like any AHA, can cause irritation, and in high concentrations, it can result in redness, peeling, and further pigmentation problems. If irritation occurs in reaction to an over-the-counter product, opt for a lower-concentration formula or discontinue use altogether and see your dermatologist for guidance.

Chemical Peels. If your hyperpigmentation requires more intensive treatment, your dermatologist may recommend a series of chemical peels. Alphahydroxy acid (glycolic) or betahydroxy acid (salicylic acid) peels are most often recommended for skin of color. Alphahydroxy acid peels are performed every three to four weeks for a total of four to six treatments. Betahydroxy peels are performed every three to four weeks for a total of three to five peels. Occasional follow-up or touch-up peels may be useful. The peels usually take fifteen minutes or so and begin with gentle cleansing of the skin. The peeling agent is then applied for anywhere between one and five minutes. You may notice a tingling, warm, or burning sensation on your skin. The peel is neutralized and then a cool compress is applied to the skin. After the peel, your skin might develop redness, whiteness, or peeling (or the skin may not have an altered appearance) for a few hours or days. The cost of each of the peels can range from $100 to $200.

Retinoids. Retinoids are derivatives of vitamin A and they include tretinoin (Retin-A) as well as its cousins adpalene (Differin), tazaratene (Tazorac), and retinol. Retinoids are particularly useful if your dark marks are caused by acne because these vitamin A derivatives are effective for the treatment of acne. Products containing vitamin A derivatives come in over-the-counter (retinol) and prescription formulations (Tretinoin, Adapalene, Tazartene). Your dermatologist can help you determine which product will work best for you. Also, as previously mentioned, your dermatologist may combine hydroquinone with a retinoid to improve efficacy in removing the dark marks.

A word of caution: retinoid products can cause dryness, irritation, redness, and even peeling. If reactions occur, either opt for a lower-concentration formula, a less drying formulation, or discontinue use altogether. Avoiding or minimizing dryness and irritation is important because the irritation could lead to further hyperpigmentation.

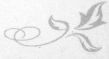

Topical Steroids. If you have a severe case of hyperpigmentation, a dermatologist may prescribe an intensive combination of a topical steroid with hydroquinone and a retinoid to lighten the skin. This type of treatment must be closely monitored by the physician to avoid side effects. Do not use topical steroids on your own (see "Dangerous Beauty," below) and do not use them for prolonged periods.

Sunscreen. To speed the fading of dark marks and to prevent further darkening of existing marks, apply SPF 15 to 30 sunblock every day, even during winter months. The best protection may be a product labeled "broad spectrum," which means it blocks both UVA and UVB radiation. Often these sunblocks will impart a whitish or purple hue to the skin, but the hue will fade into the skin within a few minutes. A frequent complaint that I hear from my patients who are athletic, very active, or who sweat profusely is that sunscreen products sting the eyes. If that is the case, consider using Waterbabies 45, which will not sting. Another common complaint is that sunscreen products are too greasy or heavy. Consider using a gel or spray formulation, which tends to be lighter and less greasy.

Dangerous Beauty

Many women of color have unknowingly used dangerous nonprescription skin-bleaching agents to lighten dark marks on the skin. Perhaps because of our quest for perfection and our greater access to discretionary income, the number of women using these products appears to be growing. Beauty supply storeowners located in major metropolitan areas that serve African, Afro-Caribbean, and African-American communities report a greater demand for bleaching products or facial fading creams. But these products often contain potent ingredients that can be harmful. Fading creams imported from as far away as Saudi Arabia, Africa, and Europe (such as Dermovate, Betnovate, Topsone, and Movate) contain powerful corticosteroids such as clobetasol propionate. All of these products are strong cortisones that can harm the skin. They should not be used without the supervision of a dermatologist. Chronic use of topical steroids can cause side effects such as skin atrophy (depressions or thinning of the skin), hypopigmentation or loss of pigment, erythema (reddening of skin), and telangiectasias (an abnormal proliferation and dilation of blood vessels). These side effects are often permanent and irreversible.

Another potential problem is the use of products containing high concentrations of the bleaching agent hydroquinone. High concentrations (ranging from 6 to 10 percent) can result in a condition that causes darkening of the skin called *exogenous ochronosis*. Although such side effects are rare in the United States, they may begin to become more prevalent as the number of immigrants, particularly from Africa and the Caribbean (countries where high concentrations of hydroquinone have been available), continues to grow.

Finally, mercury-based skin lightening products are rumored to have appeared in some beauty supply stores. These products have the potential to cause severe kidney problems and should be avoided altogether. To find out whether a product contains mercury, just read the list of ingredients or ask your dermatologist.

The safest way to reduce the appearance of dark marks on the skin is with the help of a dermatologist who can prescribe appropriate concentrations of hydroquinone alone or in combination with other skin lightening products and monitor the effects on your skin. Additional solutions may include glycolic acid products, peels, or retinoids.

Preventing Pigmentation Problems

Because of our tendency to develop skin discoloration, women of color must be particularly careful with our skin. To avoid hyperpigmentation:

• Treat the triggers. If you experience an acne outbreak or rash, treat the problem as quickly as possible with medication or preferably with a trip to the dermatologist. The longer the inflammation or irritation remains, the more likely hyperpigmentation is to occur in susceptible people. Additional conditions to treat promptly include eczema, psoriasis, and seborrheic dermatitis.

- · Don't pick your skin! It may be tempting to pop a pimple or manipulate it with your fingers. However, picking or squeezing bumps may cause further injury and hyperpigmentation—and it won't make the pimple go away any faster. A better way to treat a pimple is with spot treatments of medication as directed by your dermatologist. Alternatively, on special occasions such as a wedding or other major event, your dermatologist can inject the pimple or cyst with a small amount of cortisone. Call for an emergency appointment (but expect to pay cash for this cosmetic emergency, which is not typically covered by insurance).

- Avoid skin injury or trauma. If you're prone to pigmentation disorders, do not undergo unnecessary procedures such as deep chemical peels, dermabrasion, or laser resurfacing. If you must have surgery, discuss the possibility of hyperpigmentation with your surgeon. Application of a skin lightening agent after healing may help minimize skin darkening in the area of incision.

- Don't skimp on sunscreen. Wear an SPF 15 to 30 sunscreen every day on all exposed skin.

Myth: Dark marks can blend into your normal skin if you just get a suntan.

Truth: The sun will tan your normal skin but it will also darken the dark marks, so you will actually be worse off than before the suntan.

HYPOPIGMENTATION

The opposite of hyperpigmentation, hypopigmentation, or loss of pigment, can be just as devastating to our appearance as dark marks. In this case, melanocyte cells fail to produce pigment, causing light spots or patches to develop. *Postinflammatory hypopigmentation* can be triggered by ordinary sources of inflammation or irritation, such as a scratch, cut, burn, rash, pimple, tattoo, or surgery. It can also be caused by a medical condition such as *atopic dermatitis* (a form of eczema) or cosmetic procedures including a deep chemical peel or laser hair removal. No one knows exactly why some women of color develop hypopigmentation as opposed to hyperpigmentation, though the triggers are similar. One theory is that with hypopigmentation, melanocyte cells are damaged as opposed to stimulated.

Light marks or splotches that are classified as postinflammatory hypopigmentation tend to fade on their own after a few weeks or months. If the hypopigmentation contrasts sharply with your natural skin tone or if it covers a significant area of exposed skin, it can be just as disfiguring and troubling as dark marks.

Medical Conditions That May Occur with Hypopigmentation

Atopic dermatitis or eczema

Seborrheic dermatitis

Tinea versicolor

Pityriasis alba

Lupus

Treating and Preventing Hypopigmentation

As with postinflammatory hyperpigmentation, to speed the fading or blending in of light marks, you will need to treat the underlying cause. See a dermatologist to rule out any serious illness and to get treatment for conditions such as eczema, seborrheic dermatitis, or tinea versicolor. To even out your complexion, the dermatologist may recommend exfoliating treatments such as glycolic acid peels or products, and regular use of sunscreen. Under certain circumstances, he or she may recommend light treatments (phototherapy) to blend in the light marks. Phototherapy involves the shining of ultraviolet light on the skin, which leads to darkening of the light spots. It's important to know, however, that the normal colored skin can also become darker in color.

To prevent light marks, seek treatment for outbreaks of eczema or any dermatitis immediately, before they can cause hypopigmentation. Avoid skin injury and inflammation by treating your skin gently and forgoing any unnecessary procedures if you're prone to developing postinflammatory hypopigmentation. Finally, camouflaging the skin with makeup until your complexion evens out is a suitable alternative.

MELASMA

Melasma is a condition characterized by brown or gray spots and patches on the face. The cheeks, forehead, upper lip, nose, and chin are commonly involved. Melasma can occur in women of all ages but it seems to cluster in women between the ages of twenty-one and forty. Hormonal factors including pregnancy and estrogens, genetics, sunlight, and overactive melanocyte cells are all thought to be contributing factors. Melasma is clearly exacerbated by exposure to sunlight, with most women reporting a recurrence or flare-up during the summer months.

There are three patterns of melasma and each is based on the location of the facial pigmentation: centrofacial, malar, and mandibular. In the centrofacial pattern, the distribution of the dark areas of pigmentation includes the cheeks, forehead, upper lip, nose, and chin. The malar pattern of pigmentation involves the cheeks and nose. In the mandibular form, the pigmentation appears on the jawline.

Within the skin, the location of the pigmentation may be epidermal, dermal, or a mixture of both. *Epidermal melasma*, which is enhanced by the Wood's light, is treatable. *Dermal melasma*, which is not enhanced by the Wood's light, is located deep in the dermis and is, unfortunately, untreatable. A third, mixed type of melasma consists of pigmentation in both the epidermal and dermal layers. It is only partially treatable.

Melasma is often referred to as "the mask of pregnancy" because it occurs commonly during pregnancy. It's estimated to develop in up to 70 percent of all pregnant women, according to the American Academy of Dermatology. The condition is triggered by hormonal changes not only during gestation but also sometimes by the use of oral contraceptives or hormone replacement therapy. Dermatologists believe that the pigmentation occurs because the presence of the reproductive hormone estrogen and sunlight stimulate the production of melanin. (Darkening of the breasts, nipples, genitals, inner thighs, freckles, and moles may also occur during pregnancy, but this is not melasma.) In some cases, these dark marks fade after delivery and require no treatment. But for many women of color, melasma is a longer-lasting challenge.

Causes of Melasma

Pregnancy

Oral contraceptives or Depo-Provera (an injectable contraceptive hormone that lasts for three months)

Hormone replacement therapy

Sun exposure

Treatment of Melasma

To minimize the degree of discoloration from melasma, women of color should wear a broad-spectrum sunblock, which screens out both UVB and UVA light. The UVB portion of the sunblock must have a sun protection factor of 30 and the sunscreen must be used daily. Avoiding sun exposure by walking in the shade and forgoing the beach is a must. It's also important to wear visors or hats on a daily basis, especially during warm weather months. If your melasma develops as a result of taking birth control pills or Depo-Provera, discuss with your doctor the possibility of changing to a nonhormonal form of birth control. Women on hormone replacement therapy should also consult their physician.

There are several medications available for melasma. However, if you're pregnant, you must wait until after delivery (and after breast-feeding) before you can begin taking them. This is because of possible harmful effects of the medication on the developing baby. Once you have delivered, if the dark marks do not fade on their own (which is frequently the case), see a dermatologist. Although there is effective medication for most cases of melasma, there is no cure and melasma often recurs after treatment. That is why diligent sun avoidance is so very important. Finally, if the pigmentation of melasma is in the dermal layer of the skin, there is no effective medication.

Tri-Luma is a new topical medication used nightly for the treatment of epidermal and mixed-type melasma. Tri-Luma contains three active ingredients: hydroquinone 4 percent, tretinoin, and a cortisone in one formulation. Application of the cream will result in improvement in over 75 percent of patients after eight weeks. Possible side effects include redness, dryness, and peeling of the skin.

There are several other topical medications and procedures that are used for treatment of melasma. They are the same as those used for the treatment of hyperpigmentation, and include the skin lightening agent hydroquinone either alone or in combination with agents such as kojic acid, azelaic acid, steroids, or retinoids. The chemical peeling agents glycolic acid and salicylic acid are also useful. Finally, as mentioned, sunscreen use is essential.

Case in Point: Unmasked

When Juanita, twenty-two, made an appointment to see me, she had been struggling with the pigmentation disorder melasma for about a year. Triggered by hormonal changes during her first pregnancy, the condition caused a darkening of her cheeks and forehead. To camouflage the condition, Juanita wore very thick, heavy makeup, which was causing her to have acne flare-ups as well. Having to apply the makeup added fifteen minutes to her routine each morning, a burden and chore she did not want to bear.

To lighten the darkened skin on Juanita's cheeks and forehead, I prescribed Tri-Luma, which she applied nightly. For the treatment of her acne, I recommended an oral antibiotic, which she took in the morning and evening. I also advised her to wear sunscreen every day to prevent the sun from making her pigmentation worse. As her skin began to improve over the ensuing eight weeks, Juanita no longer needed to wear all that makeup. She also recognized the importance of daily sunscreen use. Just as she cleaned her teeth and combed her hair every day, she also applied her sunscreen. It became a part of her daily routine and ongoing prevention of the darkened patches of melasma.

VITILIGO

Perhaps the most striking pigmentation disorder in skin of color is *vitiligo* (pronounced *vi-ti-LY-go*). It is characterized by milky-white spots or patches of skin. The condition, which occurs in about 1 to 2 percent of the population, is no more common among people of color than Whites, but it is more noticeable in skin of color and more psychologically traumatizing. Vitiligo appears to have a genetic component since one in five vitiligo patients has a family member with the disease. Vitiligo typically develops in patients before they reach age twenty, but it can occur at any age. It's not contagious, nor is it cancerous.

The cause of vitiligo is not completely understood. One theory is that it may be the result of an autoimmune disorder that causes the body's own immune system to attack and destroy melanocyte cells, the cells that create brown pigment. Although most people with vitiligo are otherwise healthy, vitiligo can be associated with other disorders. For example, some patients with vitiligo experience thyroid or adrenal gland problems, anemia, alopecia, eye problems, or diabetes. Your medical doctor or dermatologist can easily screen for these disorders.

The loss of pigment in vitiligo varies from individual to individual. Once the disease has developed, its progression is unpredictable. Individual patches may enlarge, new ones may develop, or areas will repigment even without treatment. The white spots or patches of vitiligo may occur on any area of the body. More common areas include the area around the eyes, lips, or nose; on the hands, arms, or legs; and in the genital area. Genital area involvement may be particularly worrisome, but it has no negative effect on sexual response or the ability to conceive. Not every woman with white spots on the legs has vitiligo. Idiopathic guttate hypomelanosis occurs frequently in skin of color and produces small, round white dots on the legs.

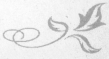

In a person of color with progressive, unpredictable loss of skin pigment, vitiligo can be devastating. The impact on self-esteem can be particularly acute in women with dark skin and in those who develop large patches of depigmented skin. People with vitiligo may find the embarrassment and stigma associated with the disease difficult to bear. The disfiguring condition can interfere with relationships as well as careers.

Vitiligo Treatments

While vitiligo is not curable, for many people there are effective treatments to bring the pigment back (repigmentation) or, conversely, to remove any remaining pigment (depigmentation). To address the problem, you will need to consult a dermatologist. You should be aware that results may not be immediate and you may need to try some time-consuming and even expensive options. In addition to the treatments, you may be able to camouflage the discoloration with concealer, special makeup, or self-tanning creams. You will always need to wear sunscreen, particularly on depigmented skin, since it has little or no natural protection from the sun and can easily burn.

Repigmentation. In order to restore lost pigment, your dermatologist may recommend one of four strategies: topical medications such as corticosteroids or immunomodulators, light therapies such as narrow-band ultraviolet B or PUVA (a therapy that combines medication and light therapy), laser therapy, or skin grafting.

Topical corticosteroids. With this therapy, creams or ointments containing potent steroids are applied to the skin twice daily. The steroids can help halt the spread of the disease and stimulate repigmentation. It's not very effective for treatment of the fingers and toes, which are difficult areas to treat in general. This therapy is most effective if you have small areas of vitiligo. It may take several months before improvement is noted. Potential side effects from long-term treatment may include

skin thinning, stretch marks, and blood vessel dilation. Topical steroids should be used only under a dermatologist's supervision.

Topical immunomodulators. There is a new class of medications called topical immunomodulators. Preliminary studies have demonstrated that these creams can repigment vitiliginous skin. Two such medications currently on the market are Protopic Ointment and Elidel Cream. One advantage of these medications is that they are steroid-free medications that do not produce the side effects caused by steroid creams (see page 164). Treatment may require several months of twice-daily application. Additional research is needed to confirm the effectiveness of this treatment and to determine possible long-term side effects.

PUVA. This repigmentation therapy combines the chemical psoralen, which makes the skin more sensitive to light, and ultra-violet A light. The psoralen is either applied topically to the skin or taken in pill form. Then, using a special box equipped with ultraviolet-emitting lightbulbs, a physician applies the UVA light to affected skin areas. PUVA is effective in restoring pigment to various parts of the body (though less effective on extremities) in about 50 percent of vitiligo patients. The treatments occur two or three times a week for months or, in some cases, years. Although sometimes covered by insurance, the treatments cost approximately $6,000, according to the National Vitiligo Foundation. Possible side effects include sunburns, freckling, and an increased risk of skin cancer and cataracts since psoralen can make eyes sensitive to UVA light. Loss of new pigment may occur over time. Pregnant women should not undergo PUVA treatment.

NB-UVB. Short for "narrow-band ultraviolet B" therapy, NB-UVB is a relatively new treatment that uses UVB light instead of UVA to repigment the skin. During treatment, a dermatologist applies a narrow-spectrum UVB light to stimulate pigment-producing cells deep in the skin. Similar to PUVA, this also takes place in a lightbulb-surrounded box. Preliminary research shows NB-UVB to be as or even

more effective than PUVA. It restores as much as 75 percent of lost pigmentation. Another benefit of this therapy is that it does not require the chemical psoralen, reducing the chance of side effects such as eye problems and an increased skin cancer risk. However, NB–UVB therapy can cause burns, pain, and blistering. Because it's a recently developed therapy, it's not widely available and more research is needed to confirm its effectiveness and determine long-term side effects.

Skin grafting. With this therapy, a dermatologist transfers skin from unaffected areas to depigmented areas. Often the result is only partial repigmentation. This highly technical treatment is also not widely available.

Lasers. In recent studies, the excimer laser has shown promise in the repigmentation of vitiligo. Patients undergo treatment three times a week. Further research on this form of treatment is pending.

Depigmentation. If the loss of pigment from vitiligo is extensive—covering more than 50 percent of skin—and not responsive to repigmentation therapies, patients may want to undergo depigmentation or complete removal of all remaining skin pigment. Clearly, this is a difficult choice for any patient, but particularly for women of color. Our skin color is part of what makes us who we are, and the decision to remove our pigmentation can be psychologically wrenching. However, it may be preferable to living with large patches of both brown and white skin. Before making such a decision you should discuss the pros and cons thoroughly with your doctor and family as well and then wait a few months to become comfortable with the decision before beginning treatment.

Depigmentation is achieved by using a potent medication called monobenzylether of hydroquinone (Benoquin). Patients apply this cream once or twice daily to the areas of skin that have brown pigment remaining. The process of removing pigment can take weeks or months. It's extremely important to understand that the depigmentation due to Benoquin is permanent. Therefore, Benoquin must never be used in any situation other than vitiligo. Furthermore, the depigmentation often occurs in areas far from the site where the cream was applied. So never use Benoquin to bleach one area of the skin. You may develop multiple white areas all over the skin. Only utilize Benoquin to complete the process of depigmentation started by vitiligo.

Side effects, such as allergic reactions to the medication, partial repigmentation, and even hyperpigmentation, can occur. After treatment is completed, however, remember that the loss of skin color is permanent. Depigmented skin no longer has natural sun protection, so the daily use of SPF 30 sunscreens and sun-protective clothing is essential to prevent sunburns and skin cancer.

Camouflage. For many patients with vitiligo, especially those with limited areas of involvement, makeup may be an ideal alternative. It's particularly useful for those women who have vitiligo limited to the face, neck, or hands. Conventional foundations or concealers may be used, although they may wipe off during the day. Many of my vitiligo patients use Fashion Fair cover toner and setting powder. Other options include Dermablend and Covermark, two waterproof cosmetic options that will not wear off as the day progresses. Have an esthetician or makeup consultant guide you in the selection of the appropriate shade and the application technique for the makeup and setting powder. If you don't get it right on the first try, don't give up. Sometimes it takes a little extra effort to get the correct shade for your skin.

Vitamins. Preliminary research by several investigators has indicated that vitamins, especially in conjunction with ultraviolet light, may help in the treatment of vitiligo. I encourage my patients to take a multivitamin daily.

Q&A Session

Q. *I've heard that cocoa butter is good for lightening dark marks. Is that true?*
A. Though cocoa butter is good for moisturizing dry skin, there is no scientific evidence that it's effective in treating hyperpigmentation. Other "natural" ingredients found in skin-care products, such as aloe and vitamin E, may be beneficial to the

skin but also have not been proved effective for treating dark marks. The safest, proven treatment is the skin-bleaching agent hydroquinone. A dermatologist can prescribe a product containing 3 to 4 percent hydroquinone to treat your hyperpigmentation. You might also use cleansers or lotions containing glycolic acid to exfoliate the skin and even its tone.

Q. *I have freckles on my face and shoulders. How can I get rid of them?*

A. Freckles are simply small circular areas of increased pigmentation. You probably have an inherited tendency to develop them and the sun will often make more develop. While freckles are not harmful and will never become cancerous, many women wish to remove them to improve their appearance. You have several options. Make an appointment with a dermatologist to determine what the best treatment is for you. You can either have the freckles removed permanently or, if you have an abundance of freckles, they can be diminished. To remove them, your dermatologist might recommend cryosurgery, a treatment that uses liquid nitrogen to freeze the pigmented skin, causing freckles to disappear (the liquid nitrogen can cause a white discoloration of the skin). Or, the physician might suggest electrodesiccation, a procedure in which an electric needle is applied to the freckle to destroy the pigment (but a dark spot could develop).

If your freckles are extensive, you may want to diminish their appearance by trying microdermabrasion, a cosmetic technique that uses fine crystals to exfoliate the uppermost layers of skin. This technique, however, carries risks for women of color, including scarring and increased pigmentation. Discuss the pros and cons with a dermatologist with experience treating skin of color. I don't recommend trying natural remedies to lessen the appearance of your freckles as any untested agent can potentially irritate the skin and increase your sensitivity to pigmentation disorders. Women with a history of keloid scarring should not have freckles removed.

Q. *I have suffered with vitiligo for many years. Treatment has been somewhat effective but the condition has made me terribly self-conscious. What can I do?*

A. You don't have to suffer with the problem alone. First, make sure you've received the latest treatment by visiting a dermatologist. New therapies, such as narrow-band ultraviolet B (NB-UVB), may be more effective in restoring pigmentation than older treatments such as topical corticosteroids. You can also use your appointment time to discuss camouflaging techniques such as using concealer, self-tanning creams, and makeup to lessen the appearance of your condition. It might help to visit a makeup artist at a spa or makeup counter to get additional tips. Improving the appearance of your depigmented skin may take some time, effort, and patience on your part, but the effect on your self-esteem will be worth it.

Once you've sought the latest treatment, you might also want to consider joining a vitiligo support group. The disfiguring nature of vitiligo can be quite difficult to cope with alone. Discussing your concerns about your appearance, treatment options, relationships, and career issues with others can be enormously beneficial and informative. To locate a support group in your area, contact the National Vitiligo Foundation, 611 South Fleishel Avenue, Tyler, Texas 75701; (903) 531–0074; www.nvfi.org/support.htm.

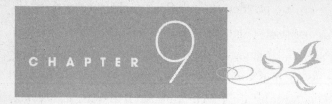

CHAPTER 9

ACT AGAINST ACNE

Acne is one of the biggest challenges to women of color who seek clear, glowing complexions. Though acne pimples are often associated with teenage skin, many adult women complain about unattractive whiteheads, blackheads, pimples, and large acne cysts. Some women of color have acne most of their lives while others develop it for the first time in their twenties or thirties.

It's quite common for acne to develop during adulthood. Most of my acne patients are adult women in their twenties, thirties, and forties. Usually by age fifty-five, acne subsides. At any age, acne takes patience and care to treat. Severe, persistent acne is more than just a cosmetic problem: not only can it lead to scarring, but it can negatively impact self-esteem and our well-being.

As a woman of color with acne, you may also face a double whammy if hyperpigmentation—skin darkening in spots or patches—occurs in response to an acne outbreak. Because of its reactive nature, the melanin in our skin may respond to acne by producing excess pigment. When that occurs, dark marks develop. The combination of dark spots and acne pimples or cysts can be very unsightly, compounding the psychological impact of the condition. Often dark marks remain even after the acne flare-up is treated, and those marks may take months, if not years, to fade.

Whether you have mild or severe acne, you'll be pleased to learn there are multiple effective treatments for the condition. With several topical and oral prod-ucts to choose from, you can successfully treat an acne outbreak. But you'll also need to learn how to cleanse and care for your acne-prone skin and prevent flare-ups from occurring in the first place. (See "Your Acne Skin-Care Program," page 191). Preventing acne, and treating it and any dark marks that occur promptly, are key steps to keeping your skin of color smooth and blemish-free.

WHAT IS ACNE?

The term *acne,* or *acne vulgaris,* applies to a range of skin eruptions that begin below the skin's surface. Beneath each skin pore lays a follicle that contains sebaceous glands that produce oil, or sebum. The follicle is also lined with a number of cells that are normally shed and brought to the skin's surface by the sebum and washed away. However, when the cells stick together instead of shedding, they form a plug or blockage. Beneath the plug, a sac is formed (known as a microcomedone) that contains dead skin cells and oil. Bacteria grow freely in this environment, feeding on the dead skin cells and oil for fuel. As the sac continues to grow, either a whitehead (known as a closed comedone), a blackhead (open comedone), or a pimple forms (see illustrations, page 172). In more serious cases, the sac will become larger (spurred on by the cells that the body sends into the sac to fight the infection) and a painful nodule or cyst will develop. Now imagine a tiny sac in the very early stage of forming. If you rub and scrub the overlying skin, the sac will break and spill its contents beneath the surface of the skin. Inflammatory cells in your body will then rush into the area and release chemicals that produce a very large, red, and inflamed bump. That's why it's important not to scrub acne-prone skin.

Many different factors contribute to the development of acne. The skin con-dition tends to run in families, so there is a hereditary component. Teenage acne is triggered by the fluctuating hormones produced during puberty. These hormones thicken the lining of skin follicles and stimulate excess oil production by the seba-ceous glands, thus plugging the skin follicle and providing food for the bacteria.

Blackhead

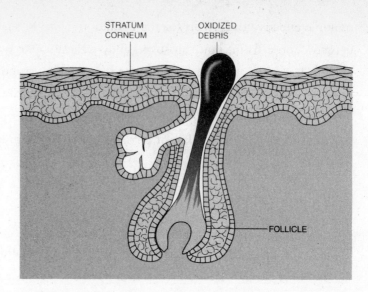

Whitehead

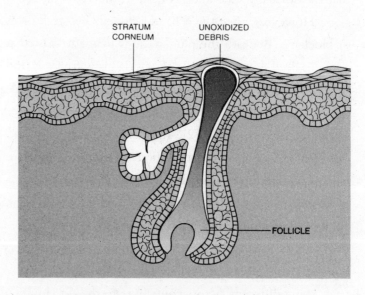

From Black Skin Care for the Practicing Professional, *1st Edition, by A. P. Thrower and H. Gambino,* © *1999. Reprinted with permission: Delmar, a division of Thomson Learning.*

Acne commonly occurs in many women during the week before menstruation and during pregnancy and the postpartum period. Acne flares may also be precipitated by heavy oil-based makeup, oily hair pomades or sprays, friction, and even stress-related hormonal changes. Although many women believe that certain foods contribute to their acne outbreaks, there's no evidence that food contributes to acne. So the good news is that fried foods, greasy foods, chocolate, soda, and candy do not cause acne!

Acne Activators

Several internal and external factors contribute to the blocked, inflamed pores that are known as acne. They include:

Hormonal fluctuations

Friction

Oily makeup

Overuse of topical corticosteroid creams

Oily pomades, gels, mousses, or hairsprays

Stress

Acne most often appears on the face, particularly in areas where sebaceous glands are abundant, such as the T-zone—the forehead, nose, and chin. Often in adult women it occurs along the jawline and lateral cheeks. But depending on the source of the acne, pimples or cysts can also appear on your neck, shoulders, chest, and back, adding to frustration and embarrassment.

Acne Types

Most of us know what whiteheads and blackheads look like. But acne also develops in the form of other more prominent lesions, including:

Papules—small or larger red or flesh-colored bumps

Pustules—white pus-filled bumps often with a red ring around them

Nodules (cysts)—large pus-filled, often painful lesions

Case in Point: Unveiling Smooth Skin

Over the years, I've treated many patients with acne, but when Barbara entered my office, she took me by surprise. She was so ashamed and embarrassed by her severe acne that she had taken to wearing a scarf tied across the lower half of her face, much like the bandits in old westerns did! At the young age of twenty-seven, Barbara was not only in hiding but deeply depressed about her appearance. Partly because of her acne, Barbara did not have a job, which only compounded her low self-esteem. She told me she simply felt too bad about herself to go out and look for employment.

During the next eight weeks, I treated Barbara with a combination of oral antibiotics to treat her infected cysts and topical medications including Benzamycin gel each morning and Differin gel each evening to clear her clogged pores. I also prescribed Lustra cream, a skin-bleaching product, to begin to lighten her dark marks. Her skin improved dramatically. By the time she came for her last visit, she was able to leave her scarf at home. We continue to maintain her on the topical acne medications as she no longer needs the Lustra or the oral antibiotic.

Myth: Foods cause acne breakouts.

Truth: There's no scientific evidence to support this belief. If you notice pimples on your face or neck whenever you eat certain foods (chocolate, fried fast foods), you may think those foods lead to breakouts. But your acne is more likely being promoted by stress-related hormonal changes that cause your skin to produce more oil and clogged pores. The foods you may tend to eat when you're stressed—sugary or greasy comfort foods—are probably just coincidental.

EVERYDAY CARE OF ACNE-PRONE SKIN

In addition to seeking treatment of acne outbreaks when they occur, you'll need to adopt an anti-acne skin-care regimen to keep your skin of color clear of pimples and dark marks. Because your skin produces the oil and cells that can clog pores every day, your skin-care routine must be consistent to keep acne under control.

Cleansing

To keep oil in check and to gently exfoliate, wash twice daily with either a medicated acne cleanser (such as one containing salicylic acid or benzoyl peroxide), with an alphahydroxy acid cleanser or a nonmedicated cleanser appropriate for your skin type. Always check in advance with your dermatologist before selecting a medicated cleanser, since some women may experience adverse effects from some of these products. I do not recommend using cleansers that contain granules, nor do I suggest scrubbing your face with rough washcloths, puffs, or sponges—these practices will only irritate the skin and cause redness and exacerbate your acne (remember that microcomedone). Instead, massage your skin gently, rinse clean with tepid water, and pat dry. If you wear makeup, be sure to remove it completely each day to avoid blocking your pores. Before going to bed, cleanse, moisturize if needed, and apply your medication.

Moisturizing

Even though oil is part of what causes acne, you may still need to moisturize your acne-prone skin. As a woman of color, you have skin that is more likely to change in type in response to the change in seasons. And many acne medications are drying to the skin. To keep your skin moisturized while minimizing acne, apply an oil-free moisturizer (Fashion Fair Oil Free Moisturizer, Black Opal Oil Free Moisturizing Lotion, or for very dry skin, consider Cetaphil lotion or Olay), and depending upon your skin type, you may consider using a product that contains an alphahydroxy acid such as glycolic acid (Md Forte lotion or cream, Neostrata lotion or cream, Alpha Hydrox lotion). These acids will help unclog pores and slough dead skin cells while keeping your skin's texture supple.

Sun Protection

If your moisturizer does not contain SPF 15 sunscreen, apply an oil-free gel or non-comedogenic sunscreen lotion separately each day. Also protect your skin from the sun with sunhats, sun-protective clothing, and umbrellas. Sun exposure may make any related dark marks even darker. Certain acne medications may make your skin more sensitive to the sun.

Exfoliating

To improve the texture of your skin, you might want to use exfoliating masks once a week or so. A mask containing either salicylic acid or glycolic acid will absorb oil and help prevent dead skin cells from clogging pores. Benzoyl peroxide is another acne fighter commonly found in masks.

General Care Tips

- Try not to touch your face with your fingers, which harbor oil and bacteria. Resist the temptation to poke, squeeze, or otherwise manipulate pimples, which can spread inflammation and cause injury. Treat the pimples with acne medications prescribed by your physician instead.
- Use hair oils, gels, pomades, and hairspray *sparingly*. (You may not need to use these products at all if you wash and deep-condition your hair once a week; see chapter 4.) Avoid applying these products near the hairline where they can migrate to your forehead and face, causing acne outbreaks. Instead, limit their use to the ends of the hair and wash hair products out of your hair each week.

- Don't sunbathe. It's a myth that the sun will improve acne, especially over the long term. Wear sunscreen every day and stay out of direct sunlight by using sunhats and umbrellas at the beach or while on vacation.

- Remove makeup before you exercise. The combination of makeup and sweat may exacerbate your acne, causing an outbreak.

- Keep it clean. Wash everything that touches your face on a regular basis, including makeup sponges and brushes, which can harbor bacteria. Wash face cloths and towels frequently, and replace pillowcases, which can collect hair oils, twice a week. Wipe your work phone and cell phone clean with alcohol each week.

- Minimize stress. Acne pimples can crop up, particularly in the lower part of the face, in response to emotional stress. If you are prone to these types of eruptions, follow the cleansing tips above *and* take steps to manage the stress in your life—exercise regularly, take breaks during the day, get adequate sleep, and consider stress-busters like massage or yoga.

Take Note

If you have noticed acne combined with facial hair growth and irregular menstrual periods, you may have a condition called *polycystic ovarian syndrome* (PCOS). Ask your doctor to perform the appropriate tests. The condition is often controlled with oral contraceptive pills.

COVER GIRL: ACNE AND MAKEUP

You can still use makeup to enhance your looks and conceal your acne, but you must take care not to exacerbate the condition. A mistake many women of color with acne make is to apply layers of very thick oil-based concealer, foundation, or powder to mask acne pimples or cysts as well as dark marks. This strategy is not only ineffective—it usually looks obvious—but it can irritate your skin and trigger even more acne.

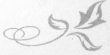

To use makeup effectively, you'll need to select products compatible with acne-prone skin. Your concealer, foundation, powder, and other cosmetic products should be water-based or oil-free. Look for products labeled "noncomedogenic" or "nonacnegenic" in order to avoid oily products that clog pores as well as potential irritants such as alcohol, lanolin, or artificial fragrances. Some liquid foundations actually contain the anti-acne medication salicylic acid (Avon Clear Finish Oil-free Foundation Anti-Acne Treatment).

To camouflage pimples and dark marks caused by acne, apply a small amount of water-based concealer a shade lighter than your skin tone. Follow the concealer with a layer of oil-free foundation and a light dusting of loose (not pressed) powder. At the end of each day, thoroughly remove all of your makeup.

If your makeup conceals pimples but not the dark marks, you might try applying more concealer, but use a light hand. Too much makeup will aggravate your acne. Talk to your dermatologist about ways to fade the dark marks—which may take several weeks to months—with 4 percent hydroquinone and exfoliating products such as glycolic cleansers or facial peels.

Myth: Squeezing blackheads or whiteheads will make them go away faster.

Truth: No! Squeezing acne blackheads or whiteheads will not make them heal any quicker and may make them worse. By picking at these blemishes, you may cause unnecessary inflammation and, in the case of whiteheads, larger acne lesions. Even worse for women of color, squeezing can cause injury and dark marks.

TREATING ACNE

Although acne can be very distressing, especially if it's accompanied by dark marks, and is not curable, you can rest assured that it's highly treatable. A variety of medications, both topical and oral, are quite effective. If you tend to have occasional mild outbreaks, you can probably treat the pimples with over-the-counter products and by making some changes in your skin and hair-care routines. For example, women who use heavy makeup or certain hair pomades will notice a significant difference in acne outbreaks by simply discontinuing use of these products. If you scrub your face when cleansing, changing to a gentler washing routine will also improve the acne. These improvements occur even without the use of medication. If the adjustments do not improve your acne, or if you have more severe acne, you will need to see a dermatologist for more potent prescription medications. You should also see a dermatologist if over-the-counter treatments do not seem to work in order to rule out any other diagnosis and to get the best treatment.

Case in Point: Stop the Steroids

Iesha, twenty-two, is typical of many women of color I have treated over the years who have used over-the-counter or prescription corticosteroid creams to treat their acne. She began using 1 percent hydrocortisone cream on her face two years ago when she developed a few pimples. The bumps cleared up and she felt that her face was smooth and soft. Not wanting to "give up a good thing," Iesha continued applying the cream religiously every day.

After six months, she noticed that whenever she forgot to use the hydrocortisone cream, her face would break out in pimples and become red and irritated. After a year her face began to break out even when using the cream on a daily basis. Iesha then borrowed her sister's prescription eczema corticosteroid cream, Triamcinolone, and began using that daily on her face. After initial improvement she began to notice red blood vessels on her face. When she ran out of the Triamcinolone, her entire face became red, irritated, and covered with pimples and she came to me begging for a prescription for more Triamcinolone. I explained to Iesha that corticosteroid creams should never be used to treat acne and that her skin was addicted to the medication. In addition, Iesha was experiencing one of the known side effects of corticosteroids—the irreversible growth of blood vessels on the skin. It would take between six weeks and six months for the withdrawal process to be completed, but I would help her through it.

I instructed Iesha to wash her face daily with plain water and then apply a thin coat of Vaseline two to three times a day while her face was going through the withdrawal process. When her face became unbearably itchy, I instructed her to apply ice water compresses or milk compresses to her face for five minutes. In addition, I prescribed two medications: protopic ointment (to be applied twice daily) and the oral antibiotic tetracyline (taken twice daily) to decrease the inflammation that occurs during the withdrawal process. The blood vessels on her face were, unfortunately, permanent. However, after three months, Iesha was finally smiling as her normal, unaddicted skin began to reemerge.

Myth: Corticosteroid creams (Cortizone 10, Cortaid, or prescription varieties) are a treatment for acne.

Truth: Over-the-counter or prescription corticosteroid creams should never be used for the treatment of acne! These powerful medications can harm the skin, especially when used for long periods of time. It may initially appear that the acne improves with the use of these creams. However, as time goes on, the skin will become addicted to the medication. This means that when the medication is stopped, the skin will become red, itchy, and uncomfortable, and many bumps will develop. So if you are using steroids for your facial acne, stop and see your dermatologist immediately so that he or she can help you through the withdrawal process.

Over-the-Counter Acne Cures

If you tend to get mild acne with a few whiteheads, blackheads, or pimples, one of the following over-the-counter products (OTCs), or a combination, might help treat the blemishes. Always check with your doctor before selecting an OTC medication so that you will use products most compatible with your skin and that will not result in dryness or irritation of the skin.

Benzoyl Peroxide. The active agent in many OTC (such as Oxy, Clearasil, and Proactive) and prescription acne medications (such as Triaz and Brevoxyl), benzoyl peroxide works by reducing bacteria (*Proprionibacterium acnes*) that cause acne. It can also assist in unclogging the pores and drying surface oil. Look for a cream, gel, or lotion containing between 2.5 and 5 percent benzoyl peroxide. (Higher concentrations designated as "maximal strength" will be too drying for many women of color.) Test the benzoyl peroxide product on unexposed skin to be sure you're not allergic or that irritation does not occur. Apply a small amount (a pea-size dot) of the benzoyl peroxide to your entire face nightly to treat the pimples that you have and to prevent new pimples from developing.

Hydroxy Acids. A member of the betahydroxy acid family, salicylic acid fights acne by exfoliating the skin, reducing bacteria, and decreasing the inflammation of acne. Dead skin cells are cleared away as well as excess oil. You can find salicylic acid or glycolic acid (an alphahydroxy acid) in many cleansers and acne washes, as well as lotions and pads. To help tame recurrent acne, use the wash once a day or twice if tolerated.

Sulfur. Another effective acne fighter is sulfur, which exfoliates the skin, clearing pores. It also fights bacteria. An over-the-counter product will contain 3 to 10 percent sulfur. However, some people are allergic to sulfur, and it has an unpleasant odor.

Vitamin A. This antioxidant is beneficial in the treatment of acne because it treats the cells beneath the skin surface that cause pore clogging. It also encourages exfoliation. Although prescription products containing vitamin A are commonly used to treat acne, an over-the-counter form is retinol. It can be found in creams, lotions, or ointments. Like other exfoliators, retinol can be irritating to the skin, so test it before using.

Quick Fixes for Acne Emergencies

You wake up the day you have to make a presentation or attend a special event, and there it is—a big zit in the middle of your face. What to do? Don't pick at it or try to make it disappear under gobs of makeup. Instead try these tricks:

- Soak a clean cloth in cool water and hold it against the pimple for one to three minutes. Repeat the compress three times a day.
- Apply an ice cube to a red inflamed pimple three times a day to reduce the inflammation.
- Dip a cloth in a solution of warm saltwater and use as a compress. The salt will help lessen inflammation.
- Apply a small amount of water-based concealer on the blemish; apply oil-free foundation, then another layer of concealer followed by powder.
- Do not use toothpaste, mouthwash, or baking soda to treat your pimples. Instead ask your doctor if a dab of benzoyl peroxide will help your pimples or if an injection of cortisone may be in order.

Prescription Problem-Solvers

Acne that does not respond to over-the-counter topical products might be best treated with stronger prescription treatments. Your dermatologist will be able to effectively treat all types of acne, including the pus-filled papules, larger acne nodules, or painful acne cysts. Prescription acne medications range from topical or oral antibiotics to hormonal therapies to Accutane. By relying on your physician, you'll find the most appropriate treatment for, and prevention of, acne flare-ups. But be patient—depending on your condition, it may take several weeks or even months to see improvements. Also be responsible. Use the medications exactly as directed by your physician. (Do not skip dosages unless instructed by your doctor.)

Antibiotics. To kill the bacteria that cause and exacerbate acne pimples and cysts, your dermatologist may prescribe topical (creams, solution, gels, pads) or oral antibiotics. These medications are also effective in decreasing inflammation. Since antibiotics address only the bacterial component of acne, they are usually prescribed in combination with other acne medications. Oral antibiotics are in general more effective than the topical variety. Many people with acne will need to take oral antibiotics for many months or even years because they simply control but do not cure acne.

There are side effects associated with the oral antibiotics, including upset stomach, dizziness, headache, increased sun sensitivity, yeast infections, rash, and hives. Another word of caution: the use of oral antibiotics by women who are on birth control pills could make the pill less effective, subjecting women to the risk of an unwanted pregnancy. Discuss with your doctor the use of a second form of contraception when taking oral antibiotics. Also, don't forget to wear sunscreen to avoid the risks of sunburn when taking oral antibiotics. The following is a list of some of the more common antibiotics used for the treatment of acne.

Topical Antibiotics

Clindamycin (Cleocin T solution, gel, lotion, or Clindagel)
Erythromycin solution, gel (Emgel or A/T/S solution)
Sulfacetamide/sulfur lotion (Klaron or Novacet lotions)
Clindamycin and benzoyl peroxide combination gel (Benzaclin, Duac)
Erythromycin and benzoyl peroxide combination gel (Benzamycin)

Oral Antibiotics

Tetracycline—250 to 500 mg bid
Minocycline—50, 75, 100 mg qd–bid (Minocin, Dynacin)

Doxycycline—50, 75, 100 mg qd–bid (Monodox, Doryx)

Erythromycin—250–500 mg bid

Trimethoprim/Sulfamethoxazole ds qd–bid (Bactrim, Septra)

*(mg = milligrams; qd = once a day; bid = twice a day; ds = double strength)

Antibiotics and Yeast Infections

If you develop a vaginal yeast infection as a result of taking an oral antibiotic for your acne, don't stop the taking the antibiotic. Instead, use an over-the-counter intravaginal antiyeast cream (Monistat) or ask your dermatologist to prescribe the pill Diflucan. One Diflucan pill usually knocks out the yeast infection in less than a day.

Retinoids (prescription vitamin A derivatives). Topical prescription forms of vitamin A (stronger than retinol) include Avita, Differin, Retin-A, and Tazorac. There are several different formulations of these products, which include creams, gels, solutions, and pads (see below). Unlike nonprescription vitamin A derivatives, retinoids are extremely effective at unplugging pores. Think of the retinoids as blackhead and whitehead busters. However, if after using the retinoid for three or four months you still have many visible blackheads, ask your dermatologist to perform acne surgery. That procedure involves the gentle extraction (removal) of the blackheads. (Please note that this procedure is often not covered by insurance.) Never allow a nonphysician to perform extractions because in inexperienced hands, scarring can occur.

The retinoids are often used in combination with other acne medications. Common side effects from retinoids include irritation, peeling, redness, and dryness of the skin. Some women of color complain that their skin is so irritated that it feels and looks "burned" by the retinoids. (Actual sunburns can occur in retinoid users if the skin is not protected from the sun by wearing sunscreen each day.) Improved tolerability can be achieved by instituting several simple strategies. First, make sure your doctor begins with the lowest dosage of the retinoid and prescribes the retinoid in a cream-based formula (instead of a gel or solution). Initially using the retinoid product every other day, applying a pea-size amount, and utilizing moisturizing lotions or creams before applying the retinoids can also help minimize side effects. Many dermatologists, including me, think that it is worth the trouble of finding ways to improve the tolerability of the retinoids. In addition to controlling acne and evening out the complexion, the retinoids also diminish fine lines and wrinkling of the skin! The retinoids are:

Differin cream, gel, solution, pledgets* (0.1% for each)

Tazorac gel (0.05%, 0.1%)

Tazorac cream (0.05%, 0.1%)

Retin-A cream (0.025%, 0.05%, 0.1%)

Retin-A micro (0.1%, 0.04%)

Retin-A gel (0.025%, 0.01%)

Retin-A solution (0.05%)

Avita cream (0.025%)

Avita gel (0.025%)

*A pledget is a compress or pad used to apply medication.

Azelaic Acid. This topical agent has anti-inflammatory as well as antibacterial properties, and it also treats the hyperpigmentation that often results in skin of color. One of the more commonly used brands is Azelex Cream. It is often used in combination with other acne medications.

Accutane. A derivative of vitamin A, Accutane is one of the most powerful and effective oral drugs developed to treat acne. It's indicated for the treatment of severe, cystic acne or scarring acne that does not improve with standard acne medications. Accutane decreases the production of oil by the sebaceous glands and unplugs clogged follicular canals. A short course of the drug—one or two pills a day (depending upon your weight) for five months—may be all you need to see significant improvement in your skin. For many patients, the acne does not return for many months or even years after treatment is concluded. But Accutane is not a cure for acne. (Unfortunately, there is no cure for acne.) If acne returns after Accutane treatment, it will typically be milder.

Accutane does carry potential serious risks. The most serious risk is related to birth defects. If a woman becomes pregnant during treatment with Accutane or during the first month after Accutane is discontinued, severe deforming birth defects will result. Therefore, a woman taking Accutane must not become pregnant immediately prior to taking the medication, during the five months that she takes Accutane, or for one month after taking Accutane. To prevent pregnancy, you should use either two forms of contraception at the same time or practice complete and total abstinence. There is also weak evidence of a risk of depression and suicide associated with Accutane use. Finally, dry skin, sun sensitivity, muscle and joint stiffness, and increased triglyceride levels have been reported as Accutane side effects. Although Accutane is not for everyone, I often prescribe it and believe it's probably the most effective treatment for severe acne. Only your dermatologist can determine if Accutane is the right medication for your skin. The usual dosage for acne is 1 mg/day, which translates to a range between 40 to 80 mg daily.

Cortisone Injections. These strong steroid injections will diminish large, inflamed acne cysts in short order—within a day or two. So if you have a pimple emergency, call your doctor for an immediate appointment to have that huge pimple or cyst injected. (You will probably need to pay cash for this emergency service—$25 to $85—since it is not covered by insurance.) Cortisone injections, however, could possibly trigger hypopigmentation (light spots) in brown skin or even slight depressions of the skin.

Hormone Therapy. As a woman—especially if you suffer from acne flare-ups, irregular periods, oily skin, and facial hair growth—you may want to talk to your doctor about taking oral contraceptive pills. The hormones progesterone and estrogen, which peak just before ovulation, can stimulate extra oil production in your skin's sebaceous glands. Birth control pills, which suppress natural hormones, can block this reaction, preventing acne flare-ups. My experience has been that the use of oral contraceptive pills can help to control mild to moderate acne. The more severe forms will require additional medication. Finally, hormone therapy can cause side effects (nausea, breast tenderness), so discuss all the pros and cons with your physician. The three oral contraceptives approved for use in *acne vulgaris* are Ortho Tri-Cyclen, Estrostep, and Alesse.

When to See a Doctor

Some women of color believe they can treat their acne on their own, or that acne is something they just have to live with. But you should seek the care of a dermatologist if:

Over-the-counter acne medications don't work

Your acne lesions are large and painful

You develop acne scars

Your acne causes dark marks

What to Do If the Doctor's Acne Medication Is Not Working for You

- Are you applying the acne medication to your entire face and not just on the acne bump? Only applying the medication to an existing pimple is like closing the barn door after the horse has escaped. You want to apply a thin amount of the medication to the entire acne-prone face not only to treat the existing outbreaks but also to prevent new acne outbreaks.

- Ask the doctor if you need to have your medications changed to stronger formulations or concentrations. For example, switching to the gel formulations of the retinoids or to the higher-concentration products may clear stubborn acne.

- Are you using the medications as directed or are you skipping dosages or missing the applications at bedtime? The medication will only work if you are committed to applying it as directed.
- Is the medication drying or irritating your skin and so you have stopped using it for that reason? Ask the dermatologist to pre-scribe milder products. He or she may stop the topical medications altogether and prescribe only oral medications.
- Do you continue to scrub your face? Vigorous scrubbing will prevent even the best medications from working most effectively. Cleanse your skin gently.

DOUBLE TROUBLE:
DEALING WITH DARK MARKS AND ACNE

Although acne affects women of all races, it can be more disfiguring to women of color who develop dark marks. Some women mistake dark marks for acne blemishes, but they are a separate problem and must be treated separately. After you've worked with a dermatologist to get an acne outbreak under control, he or she will likely recommend the most effective skin lightener: 4 percent hydro-quinone cream. You will probably need to apply the cream for two to three months, but no longer than six months, to fade dark marks. During that treatment period and after, you will need to wear sunscreen religiously to prevent the sun from further darkening the skin.

In addition to skin bleaching treatment, you may want to talk to your der-matologist about getting a series of glycolic acid or salicylic acid peels to exfoliate the skin and reduce dark marks. At home, you can also apply an oil-free moistur-izer containing glycolic acid to gently exfoliate the skin on a routine basis. Pre-venting further acne flare-ups is critical, so follow the "Everyday Care of Acne-Prone Skin" (see page 175) recommendations for washing, moisturizing, and protecting your skin. Avoid heavy makeup and hair pomades, and always remove your makeup at the end of the day. Try to wear your hair off your face. Keep wash-cloths, towels, and makeup tools clean. And never pick at your face!

Should acne pimples develop, treat them promptly with products or medications as recommended by your physician. The combination of regular skin care, skin lightening, and sunscreens should fade your dark marks and leave you with clearer, smoother skin.

Acne Scars

In addition to the hyperpigmentation that many women of color with acne develop, acne scars may arise and disfigure the skin. These scars, or depressions, result from the damage and inflammation done to the skin by moderate to severe acne. As your body heals damaged skin, it creates a scar. Unsightly acne scars are not likely to fade or resolve even when the acne is effectively treated, but prompt treatment will help prevent new scars from forming.

In some people of color who have acne, keloid scars develop. Keloids, which are often hard, irregular-shaped scars, may be even more disfiguring than the acne itself. Keloids rarely if ever go away on their own. To diminish their size, a dermatologist will need to perform a series of injections with a steroid solution into the keloid. Any surgical treatment may cause more keloids.

To prevent or minimize scarring, you should always have your acne outbreaks treated promptly and treat your skin gently. If you have noticeable scars, talk to your dermatologist about how you might lessen their appearance. Your physician might recommend using cosmetic surgical techniques such as chemical peels, dermabrasion, and laser treatments (including the new Nlite Laser) to exfoliate skin and minimize scars. Collagen or fat injections might also help to improve the appearance of certain types of scars. Another option is skin grafting, in which a physician removes skin from one area of the body (such as from behind the ear) to fill in depressions left by acne scars.

These treatments can be very effective in reducing scars and restoring an even, smoother texture to your skin. But because your skin of color is reactive and may respond to exfoliation techniques or grafting by producing dark marks, you'll need to weigh the pros and cons and make sure the dermatologist has performed many successful procedures on patients. Ask to see before-and-after photos and to speak to previous acne patients. If you have ever developed a keloid, however, you should not consider any form of cosmetic surgery.

TREATING BODY ACNE

Acne pimples don't just crop up on the face but often also on the neck, back, chest, shoulders, and upper arms. These outbreaks can be just as unsightly and distressing as facial acne, especially during warm weather months when you want to reveal more of your skin. They can also cause disfiguring dark marks, scars, and keloids in large areas that may be hard to treat. Body acne is treated with many of the same medications as facial acne. Often dermatologists will rely on medicated cleansers to treat these large areas. Caution must be exercised since some areas of the body are particularly delicate and sensitive. Only mild forms of the medications should be used.

If you develop acne pimples on the delicate skin of your chest, or décolletage, be sure to clean the skin daily with an oil-free cleanser, a mild medicated cleanser such as 2.5 percent or 3 percent benzoyl peroxide, or salicylic acid as directed by your doctor. Don't forget to apply oil-free sunscreen to this area when it is exposed. If you work out, shower immediately afterward to avoid sweat buildup and pore clogging on your chest. Never scrub the area.

To keep your shoulders, arms, and back clear and smooth, wash them daily and gently with a soft washcloth, sponge, or your fingertips. Again, rely on the guidance of your doctor for the best cleansing products and medications for your skin. But remember to use only the mildest forms. If pimples develop on your neck, you may need to stop using any gels, pomades, or hair oils that could seep from your scalp and hair onto your neck, clogging pores and causing acne. Also stay away from perfumes and fragrances. To prevent acne from developing on other areas of your body, avoid wearing tight-fitting clothes and shower immediately after working out. Keep all of your body skin moisturized and protected with an oil-free moisturizer containing SPF 15 sunscreen when going in the sun.

If you have large, irritating cystic acne on your neck, back, shoulders, or chest, or very persistent acne, don't attempt to scrub the lesions away or treat the problem on your own. See a dermatologist who will likely recommend a combination of prescription treatments, including oral antibiotics and a topical acne medication.

Acne and Pregnancy

The hormonal changes that occur during pregnancy may cause unsightly acne to develop for the first time. But because pregnant women and nursing mothers must avoid a variety of medications in order to protect the fetus, acne treatment options are fewer. Talk to your ob-gyn or a dermatologist about possible solutions, which may include a topical antibiotic, benzoyl peroxide, or exfoliating glycolic acid products. Please be aware that many ob-gyn physicians allow no acne medications during pregnancy.

Summary: Your Acne Skin-Care Program

- Wash your acne-prone skin with a cleanser suitable for your skin type. If your doctor has directed you to use acne medications and you have found them to be drying, you may wish to use cleansing products for dry skin. Your dermatologist may have advised you to use medicated cleansers such as those containing benzoyl peroxide or salicylic acid once or twice daily. If your doctor has prescribed acne medications in the form of creams or gels, ask for his or her okay before you begin a medicated cleanser on your own.
- Moisturize with an oil-free moisturizer with SPF 15 sunscreen.

- After obtaining the approval of your doctor, apply a small dab of benzoyl peroxide gel or cream, or other acne medication prescribed by your doctor, to acne blemishes as soon as they develop to speed healing and avoid dark marks.
- Optional: exfoliate weekly or monthly with a mask containing alpha- or beta-hydroxy acids. Obtain the approval of your dermatologist first.

CHAPTER 10

WHAT'S THAT RASH? HEALING ECZEMA

Case in Point: Living with Eczema

Susan came to my office at her wit's end. The fifty-five-year-old had had eczema since she was six months old, and it was worse than ever now. Like many eczema patients, she had also struggled with asthma and hay fever, which caused constant sneezing and stuffiness, especially during the fall months. When she came in for her appointment, Susan was covered with eczema from head to toe, but she complained mostly about itching and burning under her pendulous breasts and in her groin area. She was also concerned about squiggly red blood vessels that had developed on her chest and face. Because of her symptoms, Susan was unable to sleep at night, and the only temporary relief she experienced was from the three long hot showers that she took each day. She told me that she had been applying either Betamethasone Ointment or Clobetasol Ointment, two topical corticosteroid treatments, to her body and face for six months without improvement. The itching and burning were constant and unbearable.

The first thing I did was examine Susan's skin very carefully. What I actually found under her breasts and in her groin area was evidence of a rip-roaring yeast infection. She was also experiencing two known side effects of long-term steroid use: tachyphylaxis, or a resistance to corticosteroids, and telangiectasias, the development of small blood vessels on the skin due to prolonged corticosteroid use.

I outlined for Susan the following treatment plan. First, I treated the yeast infection with an antiyeast cream. For her eczema, I urged her to stop using the corticosteroid creams and instead prescribed Protopic Ointment, an immunomodulator (a substance that regulates the functioning of the immune system), morning and evening as well as Aquaphor emollient twice daily. Upon my instructions, Susan stopped taking the frequent hot showers, which were drying her skin, and instead limited her showers to one per day (five minutes only) using lukewarm water. I also encouraged her to take an antihistamine to control the itching of the eczema and to control the hay fever. It took about three weeks for Susan's condition to improve, but the itching and burning subsided and she was finally able to sleep.

Women of color suffer at least occasionally from dry "ashy" skin, especially in cold weather. But for many, the severe dry, itchy skin condition known as eczema is a more serious, ongoing challenge. Eczema is the second most common skin disease in African Americans. The term *eczema* describes a range of conditions that have the same basic symptoms—itchy, inflamed skin that can produce an unsightly rash, skin discolorations, and rough skin texture. Many infants and young children have this problem and eventually outgrow it. But the majority of people with eczema will be troubled by the condition well into adulthood.

Eczema can be a difficult, embarrassing challenge for anyone, but as a woman of color with eczema you probably have multiple concerns. In addition to the very dry, scaly skin, you struggle with an uncontrollable itch and accompanying skin discoloration. Itching and scratching can cause your skin texture to become thickened and leathery as well, a problem known as "lichenification." Because our melanin is more reactive to skin irritation or inflammation, either hyperpigmentation (dark spots) or hypopigmentation (light spots) can result. While struggling with an eczema flare-up, you also have to deal with the anguish of having a condition that is disfiguring and not easy to control.

Eczema appears to be on the rise, but treatments for the condition are also increasing. To cope with eczema, you'll need to work with a dermatologist to find the best over-the-counter and/or prescription treatment for your unique condition, and also adopt a skin-care routine and habits to protect your skin.

> **Myth:** Eczema is contagious.
>
> **Fact:** Although eczema causes an unsightly red rash that may even become infected when scratched continuously, it does not spread from person to person.

WHAT IS ECZEMA?

Eczema is a common condition of the skin characterized by scaly, red, itchy, and sometimes oozing skin lesions. When scratched and rubbed, the inflamed skin can become thickened, crusted, and even hardened. On skin of color, eczema may appear ashen, brown, or gray. It's also more likely to be accompanied by dark brown skin discolorations once the eczema redness fades.

Eczema is a condition that runs in families, so if a relative has eczema or the related conditions, hay fever or asthma, you're more likely to have it as well. Although many infants and children with eczema will outgrow the problem, many will not.

Although eczema most often appears on the neck, inside the elbows, and inside the knees, wrists, and ankles, it can crop up anywhere on the body. The condition is especially frustrating because the itching leads to scratching, and scratching only increases the inflammation underlying the condition. Eczema-prone skin then not only flakes but also thickens. In the worst cases, eczema lesions can ooze and scratching can make the skin bleed and become infected. This combination of

symptoms is particularly troublesome in skin of color, which is more prone to developing pigmentation problems in response to any kind of inflammation, irritation, or injury.

While eczema is treatable, it's not curable. The condition tends to flare up in response to certain stimuli (see "Itch Triggers," below) and subside on its own or when treated. The severity of symptoms varies from person to person, so your eczema may not look or act like someone else's. Paying attention to what causes flare-ups for you and avoiding those triggers is part of your eczema treatment plan.

Itch Triggers

The cause of eczema is not known, but the condition can be exacerbated by a number of "triggers"—irritants or allergens—in your environment. They include:

Excessive heat

Sweating

Irritating soaps or detergents

Dust mites

Animal dander

Scratchy clothing such as wool

Foods such as dairy products or nuts

Stress

Dry, cool weather

Roots of the Rash

Much like seasonal allergies and asthma, eczema occurs when the body's immune system overreacts to certain stimuli including foods, animal dander, or wool clothing. The body's defense mechanism responds by releasing chemicals that cause inflammation, redness, and itching on the skin. When you scratch your skin, the inflammatory response intensifies. This abnormal response to an external factor is most likely inherited. That's why many people with eczema also suffer from conditions such as asthma or allergic hay fever or have relatives with these conditions.

Eczema Types

The most common form of eczema is *atopic dermatitis*, but there are additional types.

Atopic Dermatitis. Also called *atopic eczema*, *atopic dermatitis* is the term for eczema that occurs in people who have hay fever or asthma, or in those who have a family history of hay fever, eczema, or asthma. Most often seen on the arms, legs, and neck, the red rash of *atopic dermatitis* is itchy and uncomfortable. When scratched, affected skin can thicken and become leathery or rough to the touch. *Atopic dermatitis* tends to be a relapsing condition in which rashes occur and recur in response to various triggers such as heat, sweating, coarse clothing, and even stress.

Allergic Contact Dermatitis. When the body responds to a specific substance against the skin, such as nickel in belt buckles or buttons, the condition is called *allergic contact dermatitis* or *allergic eczema*. Over time, a rash develops in the contact area. This type of eczema can be prevented by avoiding contact with the offending substances.

Irritant Contact Dermatitis. In people with this form of eczema, a rash develops in response to irritation from a product that is too strong for the skin. Soaps and cleansers are common triggers.

Nummular Eczema. This type of eczema is characterized by red, coin-shaped, dime- or quarter-sized lesions that appear on the skin. *Nummular eczema* tends to develop on the hands, arms, torso, and legs. Severe lesions can burn, ooze, and become encrusted. Like other forms of eczema, *nummular eczema* may be triggered by external factors. Without treatment, the lesions may last months or longer and can recur.

Myth: Long, hot baths or showers will make eczema symptoms improve.

Fact: Although long, hot baths or showers may feel good, at least temporarily, they serve to further dry the skin, exacerbating eczema. If you have eczema-prone skin, take brief showers and use cool or lukewarm water for showers or baths.

DAILY ECZEMA SKIN CARE

As you have learned, people with eczema have dry, itchy skin. To avoid a flare-up of eczema and resulting skin discolorations that can occur in response to eczema in skin of color, you need to be extra gentle with your skin.

Cleansing. Wash only once a day, unless you wear makeup, to avoid excessive drying of your skin. Always cleanse with mild, nonirritating cleansers (such as Dove Daily Hydrating Cleansing Cloths, Cetaphil Gentle Skin Cleanser, Olay Sensitive Skin, Neutrogena Extra Gentle Cleanser) and lukewarm water. If your skin gets extra dry in winter, switch to a cleanser with gentle emollients (Aveeno Moisturizing Bar for Dry Skin, Eucerin Gentle Hydrating Cleanser, Olay Complete Moisturizing Body Wash for dry skin). Do not use cleansers containing granules, loofahs, or rough cloths, which may only irritate your skin further. Limit your baths or showers to five minutes and use lukewarm or cool water. Gently pat skin dry.

Moisturizing. Moisture is crucial for preventing excess dryness and soothing irritated, eczema-prone skin. Apply a rich cream or lotion every day immediately—within three minutes is best—after cleansing to seal in moisture. Then reapply to affected areas as needed (usually several times a day). In winter, you may need an especially protective formula such as Cetaphil Moisturizing Cream, Aquaphor, Eucerin, Vaseline, Lac Hydrin cream or lotion, or Amlactim lotion. Read labels and avoid moisturizers that contain any potential irritants such as alcohol or vitamin A (retinol), which can dry the skin and make eczema worse.

Body-Care Tips

Eczema can affect your whole body, so take the following steps to avoid excessive dryness and protect your facial and body skin.

- Take a short, warm (not hot) shower only once a day. If you work out, don't linger in sweaty clothing.
- Limit your baths or showers to five minutes.
- Use mild cleansers that do not contain fragrance or other irritants.
- Apply moisturizer to damp skin within three minutes of showering to lock in moisture.
- During the winter months, dress in layers and choose soft fabrics like cotton.
- Change sheets and pillow covers frequently to minimize dust mites and cover mattresses with mattress pads.
- Use liquid detergents that are preservative-free.
- Provide double protection for your hands with rubber as well as cotton gloves during "wet work"—housework, washing the car, and so on. Rubber gloves are a necessity for all wet work. When you use them, wear cotton gloves underneath to protect your hands from the rubber and to absorb the perspiration.
- Use a humidifier to counter dry indoor heat or distribute plants around the room.
- *Don't scratch!* Scratching dry skin will only irritate it and may make eczema rashes worse. Remember: irritated skin of color is prone to discolorations. Instead of scratching, moisturize the dry skin, or if itching is irresistible, apply an ice water or milk compress to the skin for five minutes.

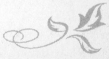

Myth: Eczema is caused by dirt or poor hygiene.

Fact: Our immune system's response to certain triggers—heat, sweat, coarse clothing—is what's behind eczema. Poor hygiene or dirty skin is not a contributing factor, and excessive washing may even make eczema worse.

TREATING ECZEMA

Once eczema flares, treating it promptly is key to not only eliminating the itch but also avoiding any further dark or light marks that might result from scratching. You have many different options for treating eczema, including both over-the-counter products and new prescription medications. Since eczema can be difficult to control and psychologically distressing, I recommend that you work closely with a dermatologist to identify the best solution or combination of solutions for your skin.

The first line of defense for many people with eczema is an over-the-counter corticosteroid cream or ointment such as Cortaid or Cortizone 10. All cortisone products are anti-inflammatory and help many people with mild eczema. Dermatologists instruct patients to apply the cortisone to the affected area or areas of skin twice daily for a two- to three-week period. However, if a nonprescription steroid cream or ointment does not relieve your symptoms in that period, it's time to see your physician and ask about the suitability of stronger medication. They include the following.

Prescription Topical Corticosteroid Preparations

A more potent version of over-the-counter anti-inflammatory products may be all you need to stop the itch and control the eczema flare-up. These prescription items come in different strengths and formulations (see box, page 201). Topical corticosteroids are divided into three categories, which include high, mid, and low potency. For thin, delicate skin such as that on the face, eyelids, and genitals, only low-potency steroids should be used and then for only a two-week period. High-potency steroids, which are the strongest and most likely to produce side effects, must be used only for a two-week period, never longer and never on areas where the skin is thin. Mid-potency steroids may be used for slightly longer periods of time. The formulations of the corticosteroids include creams, ointments, gels, lotions, foams, and oils. As with nonprescription creams, you apply the product to the affected skin only twice a day. These products can, however, cause side effects such as irreversible skin thinning and blood vessel growth if used over an extended period of time, such as for months or years. Follow your dermatologist's instructions and let the doctor know immediately if side effects develop or if the steroids are not working so that the potency can be changed. Also, when the eczema has cleared, stop the cortisone since continued use not only will harm the skin but the cortisone will not be effective the next time your eczema flares up.

Topical Corticosteroid Potencies

HIGH POTENCY: Ultravate, Temovate, Diprolene, Cormax, Psorcon
MID POTENCY: Elocon, Cutivate, Westcort, Synalar, Dermatop
LOW POTENCY: Aclovate, Desowen, Hydrocortisone 2.5 percent, Tridesilon

Systemic Corticosteroids

If an eczema flare-up is severe, your doctor may recommend an oral steroid medication (Prednisone, Methyprednisolone) or a steroid injection (Aristocort, Kenalog). Systemic corticosteroids attack inflammation from the inside. This treatment may be used to get a rash under control but not as a long-term solution because of potential side effects. Long-term side effects may include the development of hypertension, diabetes, bone thinning, and weight gain, to name just a few. Also, when you stop using the oral medication, the eczema may flare up again.

Tar

To control eczema, your physician may recommend an old-fashioned treatment containing tar. The products used most often are tar liquids for the bath. These include Balnetar bath or Zetar emulsion and tar creams such as Fototar cream or Estar gel. While the mechanism is not well understood, taking a tar bath for ten minutes, for example, may help decrease the inflammation and stop the itching of eczema. Although tar creams or gels used overnight are messy, they often help eczema, especially when your improvement from the use of other medications appears to be at a standstill. The tar therapy usually lasts for four to six weeks. I've found it to be worthwhile for many of my patients.

Phototherapy

With this therapy, a physician instructs you to stand in a light box equipped with special ultraviolet B–emitting bulbs. The UVB rays (similar to the sun's rays but without the heat) treat the eczema. Phototherapy treatments typically are given three times per week in the doctor's office, with the actual time in the light box ranging from five to twenty minutes. Possible side effects include sunburns or tenderness of the skin. (People who are claustrophobic should avoid this treatment.)

Topical Immunomodulators (TIMS)

Recently approved by the Food and Drug Administration, the topical immunomodulators known as Protopic ointment (tacrolimus) and Elidel cream (pimecrolimus) address the underlying immune system response to irritants or allergens. These prescription medications work by altering immune response. That means they counter not only symptoms but also the underlying causes of eczema. TIMS appear to be very effective in studies, reducing or eliminating symptoms in up to 80 percent of patients. This new class of drugs is as beneficial as steroids but without the potentially harmful side effects. I prescribe topical Protopic ointment or Elidel cream for my patients, and the results have been quite good. Side effects have included temporary stinging or burning of the skin.

Oral Antibiotics

If your eczema is oozing or if the skin is broken, an oral antibiotic can reduce the bacterial infection and hasten healing. One of the commonly used antibiotics for skin infections is prescription Keflex (cefalexin). It's usually prescribed four times per day for seven to ten days. Remember, when you begin a course of antibiotics for an infection, it's important to complete the course.

Antihistamines

Oral antihistamines help to alleviate the itching associated with eczema by reducing histamine levels that are often elevated in people with eczema. Benadryl and Atarax are the most commonly used antihistamines, although other antihistamines such as Zyrtec, Allegra, and Claritin are also often prescribed.

Quick Itch Reducer

If you have a mild flare-up of eczema, you can reduce inflammation and itching by applying a cool compress (a washcloth saturated with cold milk or ice water) to the skin. Then apply a dab of an emollient or moisturizer. This is a quick and effective solution if you develop itchy eczema when you're on the go and don't have your medicine on hand.

Case in Point: Getting Rid of the Rash

Hilda, a twenty-six-year-old woman who had had eczema all of her life, came to me with a severe outbreak. She was chilled, itchy all over, and extremely uncomfortable. Hilda's skin was dry, flaky, uneven in color, and quite thickened from her constant rubbing and scratching. Further compounding her condition, she had difficulty sleeping. Hilda's eczema was making her miserable.

Given the severity and extent of her disease, I decided to prescribe a few treatments. In addition to the high-potency cortisone ointment, Ultravate, morning and night for application on the thickened areas of skin, I prescribed cortisone pills (Prednisone) in tapering dosages for a two-week period. I also recommended that she apply Protopic ointment twice daily on day 15 so that we would have an effective medication when the steroid was discontinued. Finally I prescribed the anti-itch pill Zyrtec to be taken once daily.

When Hilda returned to my office three weeks later, her skin was much improved. The itching had diminished sufficiently so she could sleep through the night. We continued the Protopic ointment as well as the emollient, Aquaphor, twice daily. To prevent further flare-ups during the winter months, I suggested that Hilda alter her bathing habits, obtain a humidifier for her bedroom (to increase the moisture in the air), and avoid wearing wool clothing.

ITCHING, RASHES, AND DARK MARKS

In women of color, eczema can unleash a chain reaction of problems for the skin. Dry, itchy skin leads to scratching and further inflammation, which leads to possible discoloration. A thick, red rash can be unsightly enough without dark spots or light patches to go with them. What's worse is that the hyperpigmentation that results from eczema can be quite dramatic.

If you already have some discoloration, you must first get the eczema under control with either over-the-counter or prescription medications. Then see your dermatologist about lightening darks marks with hydroquinone bleaching creams. However, hydroquinone can irritate eczema-prone skin, so be sure to patch-test the hydrocortisone on a small area of skin first.

If, on the other hand, you have developed light marks that are either white or pink in color, your dermatologist will not have many therapeutic options. The most important strategy is to treat the eczema, remove the inflammation, prevent scratching, and wait for the color to blend in. The blending-in process may require months or years. In the meantime, you need to take every precaution to prevent another eczema flare-up. Each day, thoroughly moisturize your skin and avoid any potential irritants such as cleansers, detergents, and wool clothing. Minimize time spent in dry, hot environments and consider getting a humidifier. Also, be alert to allergens like animal dander or dust mites. Resist the temptation to scratch by carrying moisturizer wherever you go and remind yourself that chronic scratching can wreak havoc on skin of color.

The progression of your eczema may be hard to predict because flare-ups tend to come and go. If for any reason moisturizing and using medications ceases to keep your itching and rash in check, see your dermatologist right away. You may need to switch medications or reevaluate your treatment plan. The sooner you do this the better, to prevent unnecessary suffering and worsening of the condition. Prompt treatment will help keep your skin smooth, clear, and soft.

Q&A Session

Q. *Can alternative remedies such as evening primrose oil work to relieve itching?*
A. Although some people may find alternative or complementary treatments beneficial, there's no scientific evidence to support the notion that these remedies actually work in treating eczema. Before you experiment with any form of alternative treatments, consult your dermatologist. Certain alternative remedies may interfere with medications. Also, an essential oil such as evening primrose may irritate your already inflammation-prone skin. As a woman of color, you need to be especially careful about not irritating your skin, since irritation can result in further hyperpigmentation (dark marks) or even hypopigmentation (light marks). A better strategy is to keep your skin hydrated with nonirritating moisturizers between eczema outbreaks and to seek proven treatments when rashes develop.

Q. *Should I get tested for allergies?*

A. Maybe. Eczema is associated with hay fever, a very common allergy. However, the two conditions are distinct—one involves the skin, the other involves the upper respiratory system. Talk to your physician. If you suspect you are allergic to a particular substance such as nickel (in buttons, belts), fragrances, preservatives, or various foods (dairy products, nuts, berries), an allergist or dermatologist can help you determine if this is the case. By conducting either a skin patch test or a blood test, the allergist or dermatologist may be able to pinpoint an allergic source of your eczema. However, in most cases, eczema is not caused by one irritant but rather your body's predisposition to inflammation *and* its response to a variety of potential irritants.

Q. *I've heard that eczema-prone skin can become easily infected. Is this true?*

A. You heard right. People with *atopic dermatitis* (eczema) are more prone to developing skin infections, including herpes and staphylococcal infections. It's important that you learn how to identify the early signs of infection and get treatment right away. Any skin infection can aggravate your eczema and potentially be very serious. For example, the herpes simplex virus can infect the rash of eczema, resulting in pain, oozing, and pus. Fever and chills are common and antiviral medication must be given in timely fashion. A bacterial staphylococcal infection can likewise produce oozing, pus, and fever. Oral antibiotics must be quickly instituted in this case.

Q. *My friend says that relaxation techniques such as aromatherapy help with her eczema. Should I try it?*

A. What works for one person with eczema does not necessarily work for another. It's a very individual condition requiring individualized treatment. While any of the commonly used relaxation techniques—deep breathing, meditation, exercise, yoga—certainly won't hurt, they may not help, either. These techniques have not been studied for their effectiveness in treating eczema. However, stress can exacerbate an eczema flare-up, so whatever you need to do to keep stress to a minimum—especially if it keeps you from scratching—will probably be of some benefit.

Q. *My eczema gets really bad when I'm stressed out. Stress is a part of life, so how do I avoid it?*

A. You may not be able to avoid stress, but you can certainly be more aware of it as it occurs and take steps to minimize it—and protect your skin. First and foremost, incorporate some stress-reducing activities, such as exercise, deep breathing, or work breaks, into your daily routine. When you are under extreme stress caused by difficulties like losing a job or a death in the family, you may benefit from counseling from a psychologist, social worker, or psychiatrist. People have a tendency not to take the best care of themselves when they are besieged by stress. Try to get adequate rest, eat properly, and avoid alcohol. Try to see a stress-related eczema flare-up as a sign that you need to take extra special care of yourself. When stress strikes, take the time to sit quietly for a few minutes each day, maintain your skincare regimen, and give your skin extra TLC. Most important, do not give in to the temptation to scratch. Use emollients or moisturizers on dry skin and get treatment if necessary.

Q. *My eczema is out of control. I've tried all sorts of remedies and nothing seems to work. This problem is interfering with my job and relationships because people don't understand my condition. What can I do?*

A. Eczema can be a very frustrating problem to cope with, but don't despair. Medical researchers are coming up with new treatments every day. In the meantime, you may simply need to find another health provider. Many family physicians can treat mild or moderate cases of eczema, but since your case is particularly acute, you will need to work with an experienced dermatologist. If you have already consulted a dermatologist and are not satisfied with your treatment, get a second opinion. Ask your family physician or friends for referrals to a board-certified dermatologist. You can also search online (www.aad.org or www.eczema-assn.org)

for a dermatologist with experience treating eczema. Be sure to ask prospective dermatologists about their background and success in treating eczema patients, particularly patients of color. Don't settle for a physician who isn't sensitive to the scope of your problem. If you also suffer from known allergies, you may need to work with an allergist to get the best results from treatment. With the aid of these experts, you can make changes in your skin-care routine and lifestyle that will help keep your eczema in check. But you will need to be patient—trial and error is the only way to find a solution that works for you and even the most effective treatments take time to produce satisfactory results.

Also, don't neglect the psychological aspect of living with eczema. A support group may be just what you need to cope with work or relationship problems. To find one, ask you family physician, dermatologist, or local hospital for a referral, or consider starting one yourself. In some cases, a mental health professional can also be an important part of your healing.

Summary: Your Eczema Skin-Care Program

- Wash your skin once a day with a mild, nonirritating cleanser. Switch to moisturizing cleanser in cold weather.
- Apply emollients or lotion to damp skin. Reapply as needed throughout the day.
- Avoid excessive heat, humidity, and sun exposure.
- During severe flare-ups, consider bathing for only two minutes.
- Trim nails to prevent scratching. Avoid rubbing the skin, which is just as harmful as scratching.
- Optional: when eczema is not active and skin feels healthy, you might patch-test a skin lightening cream. If you have no adverse reaction to the cream, you may use it to lighten dark marks.

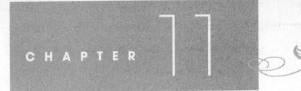

CHAPTER 11

SCAR WARS

All women of color have scars, reminders that our skin is vulnerable and is exposed to potential injury throughout our lives. Most of the time, scars develop and diminish as part of the skin's natural healing process. But among Brown women, a more disfiguring type of scar is more common. Known simply as "keloids," keloidal scars result from the same types of injuries other scars do—cuts, burns, surgery—but they behave quite differently. Keloids tend to be large, hardened scars that extend beyond the boundaries of the original wound. They, in a sense, take on a life of their own and can grow uncontrollably for weeks, even months, without treatment. These scars are one of the most disfiguring skin problems that affect Browns more often than Whites.

If you have ever had a keloidal scar, you know that it's more than a minor cosmetic problem. Keloids can grow quite large and may become painful and itchy. They can decrease the range of motion if they are located on or around a joint. If a keloid develops in a visible area, such as on the earlobes or chest, as they often do, these scars can be particularly devastating. Because they can, in some cases, be unsightly and difficult to treat, keloids can be harmful to your self-image and have a negative impact on other aspects of your life as well.

Despite these facts, there are options for women of color who are prone to developing keloids. Effective treatments are available and more are in development.

Although you cannot completely eliminate a keloidal scar once it has formed, with the help of a dermatologist you can diminish its appearance substantially and learn what you need to do to avoid future scars.

Fact: Keloidal scarring occurs in all races but it's between three and eighteen times more common in Blacks than in Whites.

What Types of Injuries Lead to Keloids?

Cuts, scrapes, or burns

Nicks from shaving, waxing, or plucking hair

Ear and other body piercings

Tattoos

Common skin conditions that cause scars, such as acne or chicken pox

Surgery

KELOIDS VS. NORMAL SCARRING

A scar is your body's way of healing an injury caused by a scrape, burn, piercing, surgery, or other type of wound. The size and duration of a scar may depend on the seriousness of the injury, the wound's location, and even your age. Young children's scars tend to be less apparent over time, and it is unusual for babies or toddlers whose ears are pierced to form keloidal scars. In adults, scars may heal with redness or a discoloration initially and then gradually fade over time. Because, as women of color, we have a tendency to develop pigmentation disorders, our scars may be slightly darker or lighter than the surrounding skin and never completely blend in. We're also more prone to scarring and discoloration if we have skin diseases like acne, eczema, or folliculitis. Although most of our scars are level with the surface of the skin (normal scarring), some may be depressed or atrophic, thus creating a crater in the skin. Still others may be raised, as in hypertrophic scars or keloids.

A keloidal scar is distinct from normal scarring in a few ways. Keloidal scars tend to be large, often growing to the size of a grape or lemon or bigger. Unlike normal scars, they extend beyond the borders of the original injury and above the skin's surface. They are often hard, have a smooth surface, and are an irregular shape (the word *keloid* means "claw" or "crablike"). They are usually hairless and sometimes shiny. The color of the scars can range from pinkish red to purple to almost black. The skin surrounding the keloid may also darken or turn gray.

In addition to being disfiguring, the scars can hurt, become itchy, and even become infected. Keloids most often appear on the earlobes, face, chest, or back, but they can appear anywhere. In most cases, they are the results of injury or trauma to skin, but I've treated patients who've developed keloids without any known injury or with an injury so minor they didn't notice it.

The cause of keloids is not completely understood, but they do tend to run in families. Why are they more common in Blacks? As a wound heals, new collagen—a protein that gives the skin its firmness and elasticity—is made and old collagen is broken down. In a person who has keloids, there appears to be some imbalance between collagen's production and its breakdown. The skin produces more collagen than is needed and fails to break down collagen, leaving the individual with excess scar tissue. This abnormal wound healing may be more common in Blacks because research indicates we tend to have larger fibroblasts, which are the cells in the dermal layer of skin responsible for making collagen. In addition to being large, the fibroblast cells contain more than one nucleus and other irregularities when compared to nonkeloid skin cells.

Unlike normal scars, once keloids develop, they can grow uncontrollably and unpredictably, and they often recur after treatment. If you have ever had a keloid scar, the chances of getting another one is not guaranteed but are very high.

Myth: All Blacks have keloids.

Fact: Though Blacks are three to eighteen times more likely to develop keloidal scars than Whites, it's not a universal trait.

Scar Types

- *Normal.* A mark, level with the surface of the skin, left by the healing of injured tissue. A normal scar may initially appear red or silvery but usually fades with time.
- *Atrophic.* A scar that is depressed beneath the level of the skin. That depression may be slight or rather large or craterlike.
- *Hypertrophic.* A hypertrophic scar is a raised, firm scar that develops within the boundaries of the skin's wound. It may be lighter or darker than the normal skin tone. Hypertrophic scars do not typically diminish without treatment.
- *Keloid.* A large, raised, often hardened scar that grows outside of the boundaries of the original wound. It may be red or purplish in color and will not reduce in size without treatment.

PREVENTING KELOIDS

If you've ever had a keloid or have family members who are prone to the condition, you should take extra-special care of your skin. Any type of cut or scrape could develop into a keloid, so you'll need to try to avoid injuring your skin and learn to care for wounds properly and promptly. To protect your keloid-prone skin:

- Treat cuts or burns promptly. (See "First Aid for Cuts and Scrapes," page 213). See a doctor immediately if a wound is deep enough to require stitches.
- Avoid body piercings, including ear piercings. Use clip-on earrings instead.
- Avoid shaving or nicking the skin. Use over-the-counter cream hair removers or depilatories if you can tolerate them, or waxing. Or ask your physician about using Vaniqa cream, a new product that blocks the growth of hair.
- Do not get tattoos, even in a discreet location on the body. Keloids can form anywhere.
- Avoid any unnecessary surgery such as cosmetic surgery.

- Protect your skin from injury—don't touch or manipulate pimples, keep finger-nails clipped and filed to minimize injury due to scratching, treat acne or any other skin problem promptly.
- Following a necessary surgical procedure, ask the doctor about a preventative cortisone injection(s) into the wound area.
- See the doctor immediately if you see or feel a keloid developing.

First Aid for Cuts and Scrapes

To minimize the risk of developing visible scars, always treat injured skin quickly and thoroughly.

1. Apply pressure to the cut or scrape with a clean cloth or bandage to stop bleeding.
2. Cleanse the wound by rinsing with soap and water. Pat dry with a clean cloth. Do not use hydrogen peroxide or iodine as it is harmful to healing skin.
3. Apply an antibiotic cream or ointment (Polysporin, Bacitracin) twice a day. This provides a slippery surface for the newly forming skin cells to migrate across.
4. Protect the wound with a bandage or other sterile gauze. Change the bandage at least once a day.
5. See your doctor if the cut is so deep you can see fatty tissue or if the wound gapes. You may need surgical tape or stitches to assist in healing.

How to Treat a Burn

Mild to severe burns can cause keloids, so don't ignore them. (If a burn is severe, blistering, white, very painful, or painless, you must see your physician immediately.) How to care for minor first-degree burns:

1. Cool the burned skin with running water or a cool compress—not ice.

2. Apply an antibiotic ointment or Silvadene cream once skin has completely cooled and been cleansed.

3. Cover the burn loosely with nonstick bandage (Telfa).

4. Use pain reliever (Tylenol, Advil) to lessen your discomfort.

5. See your doctor if the wound is painless, does not heal within a few days, or if you experience increased redness, pain, swelling, or fever. You may have an infection that needs to be treated.

COPING WITH KELOID SCARS

While keloidal scars are not curable, a dermatologist can offer a range of treatments to reduce their size and appearance. Successful keloid management may take some trial and error and time to work. Keloids often recur after treatment. For that reason, it's important to work with a dermatologist who has experience with keloids and is sensitive to your needs. Treatments include:

Corticosteroid Injections. Corticosteroid (cortisone) injections are the mainstay of treatment to halt the growth of keloids, to reduce the size of these scars, to make them softer, and to lessen their pain, itching, or discomfort. Dermatologists are capitalizing on a side effect of corticosteroids to treat the keloids—that is, the ability of steroids to thin the skin and therefore thin the keloidal scar. Depending on the size of the scar, a number of injections may need to be administered over several weeks or months to flatten and shrink the scar tissue. Corticosteroid injections will not completely remove the keloid. Treatment is often successful in flattening and shrinking the keloid and appears to be most effective with new keloidal scars as opposed to old keloids. Corticosteroid injections may be used prior to keloid surgery to reduce scar size, thus making the surgery more manageable. After a keloidal scar is removed, it's very important to have a series of corticosteroid injections (beginning three weeks after the removal) to prevent the keloid from growing back. If at any time after the surgery (even years after) you feel the keloid growing back, it is essential that you see your doctor immediately to have another series of injections.

Interferon Injections. These are similar to cortisone injections. Some dermatologists feel that injections of a medication called interferon into the keloid may help to reduce the size of these scars. Current scientific data do not demonstrate that interferon is more effective than corticosteroids.

Excision Surgery. I usually do not recommend surgical excision of keloidal scars. Recurrence is a common problem because surgery itself creates a wound. In fact, many studies demonstrate that the vast majority of excised keloids will recur, and when they do they are often larger than the original keloid. To avoid recurrence, dermatologists and surgeons must perform a series of corticosteroid injections after removal of the keloid. This practice can reduce the chance of recurrence by 50 percent. Radiation treatments are another option postsurgery to prevent recurrence.

Laser Surgery. A physician can also remove scars through the use of lasers. However, new keloidal scars can form in response to this surgery as well. Again, to avoid recurrence, doctors often offer steroid injections after surgical removal of scars. Other noncutting lasers may be used to decrease the redness of the keloidal scars.

Cryotherapy. This procedure involves the freezing of keloidal scars followed immediately by steroid injections to soften and flatten the keloid. The effectiveness is similar to that of steroid injection alone. There is the risk of lightening of the skin from this procedure.

Radiation Therapy. After excision surgery, a physician will apply low-dose radiation to the affected area. The radiation is applied after surgery and for several weeks following surgery. The therapy helps reduce the rate of keloid recurrence significantly.

Compression Therapy. By applying pressure to a new wound, compression therapy may help prevent recurrence of keloidal scars. This is most often used after an earlobe keloid—which is caused by ear piercing—is removed surgically. A special "pressure earring" is worn for twelve hours or more a day to prevent recurrence.

Additional Treatments. Some as yet unproven therapies include the use of silicone sheeting or gels applied to a keloid, usually at night, and kept in place with tape. Over a period of months, the silicone is supposed to help flatten the scar. Another treatment is the topical cream Mederma, which is made with onion extract. The cream is applied to the keloid in order to reduce its size. While promising, these treatments may be effective only on newly formed scars or in conjunction with surgery to prevent the recurrence of scars. This is the case with a relatively new cream, Aldara, which is applied to the skin after the keloid is removed.

Case in Point: Coping with Keloids

When Karen, a twenty-one-year-old child-care provider, came to my office, she had massive keloids on her chest, back, and arms, which resulted from a case of the chicken pox several years earlier. She was so intensely sensitive about her scars—which were about the size of walnuts—she wouldn't even let her mother see them. Clearly, the keloids were interfering with her life. She needed a health-care provider who would recognize the problem and not be shocked by her scars. She also needed someone who knew how to treat the keloids properly.

Although I could not promise Karen that her skin would return to a scar-free state, I explained to her that we could reduce the size of the keloidal scars with injections of liquid steroids. Over a period of six months, she came to my office every three to four weeks for the injections. To minimize dis-comfort during the injections, she applied a topical anesthetic called Emla one hour prior to the injection. At the end of her therapy, the keloids had become softer and flatter. Karen was very happy with the results—and she'd even felt comfortable enough to start dating.

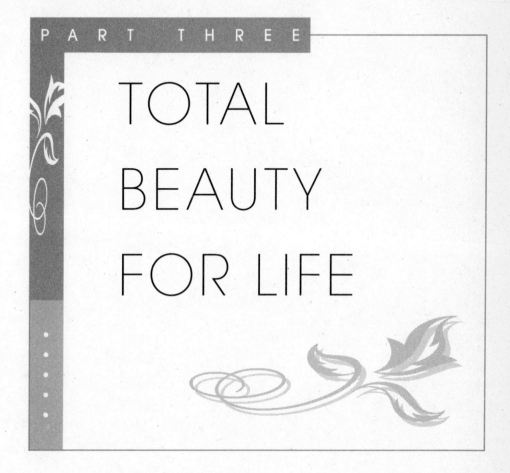

PART THREE

TOTAL BEAUTY FOR LIFE

CHAPTER 12

BABY YOUR SKIN: PREGNANCY SOLUTIONS

As a woman of color you can expect several changes in your skin, hair, and nails during pregnancy. Some of these changes are quite positive—glowing skin and thicker, more lustrous hair. But other potential developments, including excessive perspiration, darkened skin, brittle nails, and stretch marks, to name a few, are less desirable. All women experience the effects of high hormonal levels and other changes during the nine months before their baby arrives. For women of color, however, problems such as the "mask of pregnancy" and unexpected skin growths are often much more noticeable and distressing.

In addition to concerns about appearance during pregnancy, you, like many expectant moms, are probably worried about your unborn child's health and well-being. You may have questions regarding the use of hair and nail products, and how chemicals in products commonly used by women of color may affect the fetus. You may also be wondering what medications are safe and what you'll need to avoid in order to protect your baby from harm. From the perspective of a mother and woman of color dermatologist, I offer you practical answers that will calm your fears.

Many of the pregnancy-related skin, hair, and nail changes you experience are temporary and will subside on their own after your baby is born. In the meantime, there are several steps you can take to minimize your discomfort during pregnancy and maximize the "glow" of this special time in your life. To look your best, I recommend that you learn as much as you can about what's happening to your body, follow a daily skin-care regimen that adapts to pregnancy-related changes (see page 230), and attend to skin problems as they arise.

Trimester Guide to Skin, Hair, and Nail Changes

While you're pregnant, you may notice some of the following differences in your appearance:

First trimester (0 to 3 months)

Shinier, more glowing skin

New moles and other skin growths (freckles, skin tags, seborrheic keratoses)

Darkening of existing moles

Second trimester (4 to 6 months)

Darkening of face (forehead, nose, cheeks, jaw), known as the *mask of pregnancy*

Darkening of skin on breasts, including the areola

Darkening of skin on the arms or thighs

A dark line running down the center of your abdomen, known as *linea nigra*

Breakouts or a return of adolescent acne

Spider veins on your face, neck, or chest

Large blue veins over the breasts

Facial hair on your upper lip, chin

Thicker, coarser hair texture

Third trimester (7 to 9 months)

An itchy rash (or itching alone) on your abdomen, thighs, or buttocks

Stretch marks on your lower abdomen, breasts, thighs, or buttocks

Varicose veins on your legs

Myth: Brown women don't get stretch marks.

Fact: Although they may look somewhat different in Browns, stretch marks are just as likely to develop in women of color as they are in White women.

GREAT EXPECTATIONS: PREGNANCY'S IMPACT ON YOUR SKIN, HAIR, AND NAILS

Among the many physical changes you'll experience as a pregnant woman, some of the most visible ones occur in your skin, hair, and nails. These outer changes reflect inner adjustments that your body makes to support your pregnancy, including increases in the reproductive hormones estrogen and progesterone. To accommodate the developing fetus, your body also experiences a boost in heart rate and blood circulation, which is in part responsible for that special pregnancy glow.

In response to these changes, your skin secretes more oil than usual, resulting in shinier skin. Hormonal shifts may also cause your hair to shed more slowly and grow faster, triggering significant changes in hair texture and volume. For some women, hormonal changes also mean stronger, healthier-looking nails. Friends and family may comment on how beautiful you look with more radiant skin, fuller hair, and more lustrous nails.

But, as you may have already guessed, not all of the pregnancy-related skin changes you experience will be welcome. Here I describe a number of common skin, hair, and nail changes that occur in pregnant women of color and what you can do about them.

Skin

Hyperpigmentation. A rise in your hormonal levels may stimulate your melanocyte or pigment-producing cells to darken the skin in several areas, including the nipples and areola, along your thighs, upper arms, and even your genitals and abdomen. The darkening may be so pronounced that you even notice a line between the skin that's brown and the skin that remains unchanged on your arms or thighs, for example. If this happens to you, don't be embarrassed: skin darkening occurs in nine out of ten pregnant women, according to the American Academy of Dermatology. It can, however, be very dramatic in women of color. *What to do*: On sun-exposed areas of the skin, such as the arms and legs, apply a sunscreen with SPF 15 daily to prevent the sun from making any hyperpigmentation worse. Wear sunhats and stay out of direct sunlight. Because the discoloration stems from pregnancy hormones, it will most likely subside on its own within a few months after you give birth.

Melasma. Triggered by hormonal changes, melasma is a condition characterized by darkening of skin on the face. This "mask of pregnancy" may develop primarily on the central facial area such as the forehead, cheeks, and nose, or in the lower part of the face including the jawline. Melasma is characterized by light or dark brown patches on these areas of the skin. It affects seven out of ten pregnant women and is often more pronounced in women of color. *What to do*: Since treatment must be postponed until after you deliver, protection from the sun is your primary objective. Avoid the sun as much as possible, especially during the summer, spring, and fall months. Wear a hat, visor, or baseball cap on a daily basis. Most important, apply SPF 15 to 30 sunscreen containing either zinc oxide or titanium dioxide, or both, every day to minimize further hyperpigmentation, and don't forget to reapply it during the day. Since melasma does not usually subside after pregnancy, you will have to rely on treatment after delivery. (See chapter 8 for more on this condition.)

New Growths and Changes in Existing Growths. Pregnancy hormones may cause new skin growths to erupt on your face and body. These include new moles, skin tags, seborrheic keratoses, and freckles. Women of color are more likely than White women to complain about moles that first appear during pregnancy. The growths are most likely normal reactions to the changes going on in your body, but they can be unsightly, and in the case of skin tags, even irritating. Existing growths can enlarge, darken, and become irritated. *What to do*: Since it is difficult to distinguish normal growths from abnormal ones, see your doctor or dermatologist. (For some general tips on what may be suspicious, see "Pregnancy Moles or Melanoma?" page 228). Finally, you can have moles, keratoses, and skin tags easily removed after pregnancy.

Acne. Pregnancy hormones may cause an eruption of acne for the first time or a return of adolescent acne. You may notice small pimples, blackheads, whiteheads, or larger acne lesions on your face, chest, shoulders, back, and other parts of the body. In women of color, acne is a particular problem because it can trigger hyperpigmentation. *What to do*: Because you are pregnant and must be careful about any medications you use or come in contact with, I do not recommend that you try to treat your acne. You can, however, wear an oil-free SPF 15 to 30 sunscreen daily to help minimize the risk of hyperpigmentation. Limit the amount of hair oils or pomades you use since these can migrate to the face and exacerbate acne. Thoroughly remove makeup each day and cleanse gently.

Excessive Perspiration. Many pregnant women notice they sweat more. This occurs because of an increase in your basal metabolic rate. Too much sweating is not only embarrassing if you frequently soak through clothes, but it is potentially unhygienic. *What to do*: Drink water frequently throughout the day. Shower or bathe more than once a day if necessary. Carefully and thoroughly dry underneath body fold areas, such as your breasts or the abdominal area. Apply absorbent powders under the breast, arms, and in the abdominal fold area. Use antiperspirants and deodorants. Dress in layers of light cotton or other natural-fiber materials that absorb perspiration. Wear loose clothing, avoid tight elastic bands, and allow the air to circulate in the body fold areas as much as possible. Avoid excessive heat indoors or out.

Yeast Infections. Because you're sweating more and you'll probably experience significant breast enlargement and weight gain during pregnancy, you may develop yeast infections under your breasts or in the groin area. You'll know this is happening if you develop a very itchy rash that does not go away. *What to do*: Shower daily and gently with mild soap. Dry off completely and apply absorbent powder. Wear only cotton bras, which absorb perspiration, and wash them regularly. Remove your bra at the end of the day to air out the area. Once a yeast infection develops, see your doctor for safe prescription medication.

Itching (*pruritus*). *Pruritus*, or itching, occurs commonly during pregnancy and most often during the third trimester. Although your entire body may itch, the itching is usually most prominent over the abdomen (probably related to the stretching of the skin). The itching will resolve after delivery. *What to do*: Try to avoid scratching or rubbing the skin. Apply cool ice water or milk compresses. Avoid harsh or drying soaps and cleansers. Moisturize the skin regularly. Ask your doctor if you can take over-the-counter Benadryl or use an over-the-counter hydrocortisone cream.

PUPPP. There are several rashes that may occur during pregnancy. The one that occurs most commonly is called *pruritic urticarial papules* and *plaques of pregnancy*, or PUPPP. PUPPP is a very itchy rash that commonly begins during the third trimester of pregnancy. It usually starts on the abdomen in the stretch marks. It looks like red bumps, red patches, or hivelike weals. PUPPP may then spread to the thighs and arms. The itching is very intense. *What to do*: Check with your ob-gyn to make sure that the rash is indeed PUPPP. Treat your skin gently and try to avoid scratching. Often women get relief by using an antihistamine such as Benadryl or over-the-counter hydrocortisone creams (check with your ob-gyn before taking or using any medications). For most women PUPPP will persist until delivery.

Stretch Marks. Stretch marks, or striae, occur during pregnancy because the skin is stretching rapidly, which causes damage to collagen and elastin fibers in skin. The damage manifests as dark or light lines across the skin on the lower abdomen, thighs, buttocks, or breasts. *What to do*: Unfortunately, there is not too much that you can do to prevent stretch marks. Many dermatologists feel that moisturizing your skin regularly might help. Once they've developed, stretch marks do not go away entirely, but you can minimize them. There's little you can do about these marks while you're pregnant. After you've given birth, skin creams that contain derivatives of vitamin A, such as Retin-A, may help reduce the appearance of new stretch marks. Laser therapy may be another option, but it is most effective for white or very light skin.

Spider Veins/Varicose Veins. Greater estrogen and progesterone levels can trigger the development of spider veins and varicose veins on different parts of your body. The veins over your breasts may enlarge and become blue in color. Spider veins are simply enlarged red blood vessels that appear on your face, neck, chest, or arms. Excessive pressure may cause the same problem in your legs and feet, known as varicose veins. The tendency to develop enlarged blood vessels tends to run in families and there's really no way to prevent it. *What to do*: You should wait until after delivery to treat spider or varicose veins. Many of the prominent veins on your upper body will become less noticeable after delivery. For those that persist, the available treatments include electrodessication (the drying up of tissue with an electric current applied with a needle-shaped electrode), laser therapy, and sclerotherapy (injections). Since sclerotherapy is not safe during pregnancy, it's important to wait until after delivery. In the meantime, special makeup can help camouflage veins. Also ask your ob-gyn about whether or not it's safe to wear supportive stockings to relieve some of the pressure on your legs.

Excessive Hair Growth. Also known as *hirsutism*, the growth of excessive facial and body hair may result from pregnancy hormones. You may notice hair cropping up on your upper lip, chin, abdomen, or chest for the very first time. This can be particularly unsightly if you have dark hair growing over beige to brown skin, and if the hair is coarse. *What to do*: If the hair does not bother you, leave it alone. However, if it's really noticeable and you feel self-conscious, remove it by either waxing or shaving. Do not use depilatories during pregnancy. Often the hair growth will subside after pregnancy.

Pregnancy Moles or Melanoma?

As your skin reacts to hormonal changes during pregnancy, you may develop new moles on your face and on other parts of your body. Moles that you already have may grow in size or get darker in color. These changes are typically quite normal. However, you should keep a close eye on these developments since sudden changes in moles can be a sign of skin cancer. While melanoma is much less common in women of color than in Whites, it does occur. A suspicious lesion may develop anywhere on the body, but in people of color, it more often appears on the palms, soles, nails, mouth, and genitals.

If a mole looks different from other moles on your body, grows larger than the diameter of a pencil eraser, or begins to itch, hurt, or bleed, see your dermatologist. Pay particular attention to dark spots or streaks on a single nail or toenail. This may be a sign of melanoma skin cancer.

Hair and Nails

Coarse Hair. A combination of elevated hormones and increased oil secretions from the sebaceous glands can make your hair grow more rapidly and appear noticeably thicker, longer, and shinier. That's the good news. The changes can also make your hair more difficult to manage, especially if it becomes more curly or coarse than what you are used to. *What to do:* If your hair does in fact become more oily, you may want to wash it more often—more than once or twice a week—and always follow up with a conditioner. Since hair tends to grow more quickly during pregnancy, you may want to have it trimmed more regularly, about every six to eight weeks. Style your hair as you would normally (but avoid relaxers and other chemicals during the first trimester—see "Hair Relaxers and Pregnancy," below). As always, be gentle with your tresses and enjoy the increased growth.

Nail Breakage. Many pregnant women of color say their nails are stronger during pregnancy. But others complain about weak, brittle nails that chip easily. *What to do*: Simplify your nail care during pregnancy. Keep nails clipped regularly and file them gently. Moisturize your hands daily and rub the moisturizer into the cuticles. Buff nails for shine. Try to avoid "wet work" since water will further dry the nails. Save polish for special occasions since nail polish and remover can dry nails and weaken them further. Always apply polish and remover in a well-ventilated area to avoid inhaling fumes.

Common Rashes During Pregnancy

There are a number of rashes that typically develop in pregnancy. See your ob-gyn if you develop an itch or red bumps. Depending on their origin, different types of rashes, such as those listed below, may require different treatment.

Herpes gestationis

Impetigo herpetiformis

Obstetric cholestasis

Prurigo of pregnancy

Pruritis

Pruritic folliculitis

Pruritic urticarial papules and plaques of pregnancy (PUPPP)

Polymorphic eruption of pregnancy (PEP)

Hair Relaxers and Pregnancy

If you chemically straighten your hair, you may have heard that it's not safe to continue to have it relaxed during pregnancy. This is a controversial issue. There are no studies proving that hair-relaxer chemicals cause harm to the fetus. However, to be on the safe side, most ob-gyns recommend avoiding relaxers and hair dyeing during at least the first trimester when the fetus's organs are forming. I agree with this recommendation. If you do decide to relax your hair, I suggest only one chemical treatment during the second or third trimester of your pregnancy. Because your body—including your hair—is undergoing so many changes, it's not the optimal time to chemically straighten your hair.

DAILY SKIN-CARE FOR PREGNANT WOMEN OF COLOR

Because your skin undergoes significant changes during pregnancy, you may need to make adjustments to your skin-care routine. Above all, be gentle and pay attention to your skin's needs. If your skin type does not change, you should continue to follow the suggested regimen for your skin type (see chapter 2). Otherwise, I recommend that you make these adjustments.

Cleansing. If your skin becomes more oily due to pregnancy hormones, wash it more often—two or three times a day. Because many new growths may develop during pregnancy, it's important to wash the skin gently to avoid irritating these growths or inadvertently pulling them off. Such irritation can lead to hyperpigmentation. So wash very gently with a foaming cleanser or an oil-balancing soap (Cetaphil Antibacterial Soap, Lever 2000, Neutrogena Facial Cleanser Bar, Purpose Soap). If your skin is still oily after cleansing, apply an alcohol-free toner or astringent, and use it regularly as long as it does not cause irritation. Do not apply products containing vitamin A derivatives (such as retinol) or acne medication; these products have not been established as safe for pregnant women. Be sure to remove all makeup at the end of the day.

Moisturizing. Women with oilier skin will need to apply moisturizer only if the skin becomes noticeably drier during winter months. If that happens, try an oil-free product (Fashion Fair Oil Free Moisturizer, Black Opal Oil Free Moisturizing Lotion). However, if your skin does not change substantially, continue to use the moisturizer for your skin type (see page 18). Avoid moisturizers containing vitamin A derivatives such as retinol.

Sunscreen. As always, apply SPF 15 sunscreen generously every day. If you develop oily skin, try an oil-free cream, gel, or spray sunscreen formula (Aveeno Positively Radiant Daily Moisturizer SPF 15, Ombrelle Spray, Presun 30 Gel). If you were prone to hyperpigmentation before pregnancy or notice dark marks during pregnancy, opt for a stronger broad-spectrum sunscreen (that protects from both ultraviolet A and B radiation) or sunblock with an SPF of 30 or higher. Sunscreens or sunblocks containing titanium dioxide or zinc oxide work best and might even help camouflage dark marks or melasma. (To save time, choose a moisturizer that contains sunscreen.)

Exfoliate. Because your skin may be particularly oily now, you might try exfoliating once weekly or monthly with a mild clay or mud mask designed for oily skin. (Test the mask on unexposed skin first.) Make sure it does not contain any granules, which can irritate and inflame skin of color.

Medications to Avoid While Pregnant

Below is a list of some of the drugs expectant moms should never take. Always check with your doctor before taking any type of medication during pregnancy.

    Tetracycline (an antibiotic)

    Isotretinoin for acne (found in Accutane)

    Fluconazole (an antifungal)

Minoxidil (found in Rogaine)

Acitretin (a psoriasis treatment)

HEALTHY PREGNANCY PRACTICES

To look and feel your best, you'll need to take extra special care of yourself during pregnancy. Brown women are more susceptible to a variety of poor pregnancy outcomes, including premature births, low-birth weight babies, and other complications, so you'll need to be especially mindful of your ob-gyn's advice and your health.

- Drink water. You should always be drinking eight glasses of pure water daily, but water is especially important during pregnancy. Why? Because you need more fluid to meet the new demands on your body and prevent dehydration. Drinking sufficient water will also help to hydrate your skin and keep your nails healthy.
- Eat balanced meals in moderation. It may be tempting to give in to every craving and "eat for two." But overeating can lead to excessive weight gain, which is not good for you or your baby. Undereating may also be a problem for weight-conscious women of color. To meet your nutritional needs and stay healthy, be sure to consume a variety of fresh vegetables and fruit, complex carbohydrates, and protein at every meal. Steer clear of excess sweets, fat, and salt.
- Get physical. Exercise may be the last thing you feel like doing, but it's essential for your health and your baby's health. Routine physical activity will not only help boost your energy and improve the quality of your sleep but will also help keep your weight under control (see "What You Should Weigh," page 233). Great—and safe—physical activities include walking, swimming, and other moderate routines. **Be sure to consult your ob-gyn before beginning any exercise program.**
- Rest. Listen to your body's need for sleep and leisure. Get approximately eight hours of sleep each night and take frequent breaks or quick naps if you need them.

- Avoid alcohol, caffeine, and smoking, which can jeopardize your health and your baby's health.

- Listen to your ob-gyn. Take prenatal vitamins every day and keep your scheduled physician's visits to ensure a healthy pregnancy. Call your doctor right away if you experience cramping, pain, bleeding, or any other unusual symptom.

What You Should Weigh

The weight you gain during pregnancy is a mixture of water weight, blood, fat, breast tissue, and of course, the baby. Gaining too much or too little weight during pregnancy can adversely affect you and your child. But don't worry too much about your weight: your health-care provider will help you determine how many pounds are appropriate for you to gain and what to do if you're off course. Experts at the American College of Obstetricians and Gynecologists recommend the follow general guidelines.

If you are overweight:	15–25 pounds
If you are normal weight:	25–35 pounds
If you are underweight:	28–40 pounds
If you are obese:	15 pounds
If you are carrying twins:	35–40 pounds

POSTPARTUM PROBLEMS AND SOLUTIONS

Once you've had your baby and your hormonal levels start to return to normal, you may notice even more changes in your appearance. For the most part, your skin, hair, and nails will be restored to their pre-pregnancy state—the extra oiliness in your skin will subside and nail strength will resume. However, in the short term, owing to the sudden drop in hormones and other changes, new problems may surface temporarily. Here's what to expect:

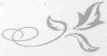

Hair Loss (telogen effluvium). Although most women will retain their longer, thicker pregnancy hair, others will have a different experience. After a long period of rapid growth, your hair may begin to slow its growth and even shed significantly. You may be dismayed to see it falling out in clumps or handfuls when you wash and style it, and even when you sleep. Postpartum hair loss is common. It usually begins three months after delivery and can last for several weeks or months. For women of color, the problem may be especially alarming because of our hair follicles' fragility and the impact of common cultural practices such as braiding. If you return to a routine of hair styling that puts stress on the hair—combing vigorously, using relaxers or hot combs, pulling hair tight into ponytails—the loss may be more significant. *What to do*: Until your hair begins to grow and shed as it did before you got pregnant, treat it especially gently. In the first six months after delivery, limit chemical treatments including relaxers and dyes. Wash your hair very gently once a week and follow with a conditioner. Comb it slowly with a wide-toothed comb beginning at the ends and working your way up to the roots. Get trims every eight weeks or so. Do not consider weaves or braids with extensions during this time as they might put undue stress on fragile hair.

Hot Flashes/Night Sweats. Though hot flashes are usually associated with menopause, they can occur in the postpartum period as well. This happens because the dramatic drop in hormones after pregnancy disrupts your body's natural temperature control mechanism. If this occurs, don't be concerned. It should subside within a few days or weeks. *What to do*: Drink water frequently. Dress in layers of light cotton clothing and avoid excessive heat indoors and out. Limit or avoid altogether caffeine and spicy foods, which can make you sweat.

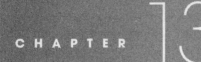

CHAPTER 13

BEAUTY AT ANY AGE

One of the best things about your skin of color is its resistance to the signs of age that are common among White women. If you consider the older women in your family, you are not likely to see very deep wrinkling or leathery, sun-damaged skin. Even if you or your female relatives do eventually develop mild wrinkling, it will probably not emerge until ten or twenty years after it has become noticeable in White women of the same age. Your skin of color simply keeps you looking younger longer.

Despite this advantage, you're probably—and justifiably—still concerned about growing old gracefully and attractively. After all, you don't want any aspect of your appearance—your skin, hair, or makeup—to make you look older than you feel. And if you happen to have a lighter skin hue, you are actually at greater risk for wrinkling and developing age spots (also known as sun or liver spots) than women of color with darker skin. As you grow older, you may also be surprised to discover uneven skin tone and new skin conditions such as *dermatosis papulosa nigra* (brown growths) on the face, which can cause marks or lesions that make you look older than you are.

To look youthful and radiant at any age, you should follow a skin-care regimen that adapts to the changes that can occur in mature skin, such as increased dryness. I recommend that you also consult a dermatologist about any developments that concern you. Your physician will be able to help you decide what to do about unwanted growths or other aging-related imperfections. As you mature, you'll also want to make adjustments in your makeup, hair, and nail care to best complement the way you look now. Finally, you should avoid any unhealthy habit or practice, such as smoking, that can age you before your time.

Your Skin, Through the Years

What you can expect:

Your 30s

Loss of the radiant glow of the skin

Dull, uneven skin tone

Slight heaviness around the eyebrows

A few new growths on the face and neck

Your 40s and 50s

Uneven skin tone owing to sun exposure and irregular pigmentation

New growths, including dermatosis papulosa on the face, skin tags on the
neck, and seborrheic keratoses on the body

A few very fine lines around the eyes and mouth

Additional pockets of fatty tissue such as under the chin and under
the eyes

Your 60s and beyond

Dryer, duller complexion owing to loss of estrogen at menopause

Darker facial skin compared to your neck or chest

Fine lines and wrinkles, especially in lighter skin

Sagging of the skin, especially in the area between the nose and the
outer corner of the mouth, or in the neck area

White spots on the legs and arms that are not signs of vitiligo (known as

 idiopathic guttate hypomelanosis)

Age (or liver) spots, only in lighter skin

Signs of Age

Our skin matures differently from White skin. Here's how:

Black Skin	White Skin
Blotchy, uneven skin tone	Freckled, uneven skin tone
Brown or black growths	Red growths
(e.g., seborrheic keratoses)	(e.g., actinic keratoses)
Dry, dull skin	Dry, rough, possibly leathery skin
Very fine lines and wrinkles	Fine and deep wrinkles
White spots on the legs and arms	Age ("liver") spots

MATURE SKIN OF COLOR

What happens to your skin as you age? In mature women of color, one of the first changes is in skin tone. Years of sun exposure and damage can begin to cause unevenness in the tone of your most exposed body part: your face. Many older women of color also notice that their facial skin is significantly darker than the skin on their neck and chest—and not just in summertime. Skin growths also tend to crop up, particularly if they run in your family. These include *dermatosis papulosa nigra* (raised brown or black growths) on the face, skin tags (raised brown or black growths) on the neck, *seborrheic keratoses* (waxy brown growths) on the body, and *angiomas* (red growths) on the body.

As you approach and enter menopause, your skin may also become dryer and more dull in appearance. This is due most likely to the natural drop in your estro-

gen levels and reduced oil production by your skin cells. If you are light-skinned, fine wrinkles will begin to set in around the eyes (crow's-feet) and mouth, and perhaps on the forehead as well. Light-skinned women may even notice some unsightly sunspots on the face and hands. Other developments might include skin thinning, loss of elasticity (sagging of the skin), and easy bruising.

Some of these signs of aging in skin of color, such as dryness and loss of elasticity, are inevitable biological changes. But, many dermatologists believe, other skin-care concerns of mature women—including skin-tone changes, dullness, and wrinkles—are probably due to years of neglect or abuse. Deliberate sun bathing and daily exposure to the sun's rays without adequate protection triggers the production of "free radicals"—unstable molecules that damage healthy cells. Over time, this process, known as "photo-aging," contributes to the wrinkling, thinning, and hardening of skin. Air pollution and cigarette smoking further barrage the skin with harmful chemicals. These factors—in addition to a toxic mix of poor diet, alcohol, dehydration, sleep deprivation, and stress—can add years to your appearance.

What Makes Skin Age?

The aging of skin is caused by more than the passage of time. A number of factors contribute, including:

Sun damage

Cigarette smoke

Pollution

Poor nutrition

Alcohol

Dehydration

Lack of sleep

Stress

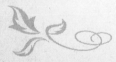

CARING FOR MATURE SKIN

What changes should you make in your skin-care routine as you age? While you can't completely stop the hands of time, you can employ strategies to minimize the impact of age-related developments on your skin. It's important to understand that the skin type you've had most of your life will change because mature skin tends to be dryer. This means you'll have to let go of cherished skin-care products and consider using ones designed for dry skin. You'll also need to adjust your regimen a bit. Here's how:

- Cleanse less frequently, perhaps only once a day. If you wear makeup, wash your face at the end of the day (so twice daily). Use dry-skin products that contain emollients (L'Oreal Hydrafresh Cleanser, Aveeno Moisturizing Bar for Dry Skin, Eucerin Gentle Hydrating Cleanser) to moisturize as you cleanse. Massage your face gently and pat dry.

- Moisturize more often. Apply a rich cream or lotion two or three times a day to damp skin immediately after cleansing. Look for products designed for dry skin (Cetaphil Moisturizing Lotion, Moisturel Therapeutic Cream, or Avon Moisture Therapy).

- Don't forget your sunscreen. If your moisturizer does not contain sunscreen, apply a cream or lotion with SPF 15 to 30, such as Lubriderm Daily UV Lotion SPF 15, Cetaphil Daily Facial Moisturizer SPF 15, or Aveeno Absolutely Radiant Moisturizer with SPF 15. This will not only guard your skin from cancer but also prevent further skin darkening and uneven skin tone.

- Utilize various forms of vitamin A. If wrinkles are a concern, consider using a cleanser, moisturizer, or eye cream made with retinol, a form of vitamin A that helps fight fine lines by stimulating collagen. Some over-the-counter products include RoC Retinol Actif Pur Anti-Wrinkle Treatment and Avon Anew Line Eliminator Dual Retinol Treatment. These can be used daily as long as they

don't cause dryness or irritate your skin. Your dermatologist may also recommend prescription-strength vitamin A such as Retin-A. or Tazorac.

- Utilize various forms of glycolic acid. To exfoliate dry, dull skin and to improve your overall skin tone, consider using lotions and cleansers containing glycolic acid.

Perimenopause, Menopause, and Your Skin

Perimenopause, the reproductive phase that bridges menstruation and menopause, typically begins in the late forties, though some women of color experience it earlier. This "change of life"—during which estrogen levels drop dramatically and menstruation comes to an end—brings about considerable changes in your skin, hair, and nails. When you enter the perimenopausal stage (typically age forty-five to fifty), you may sweat more and begin to have hot flashes. Consequently, you might also develop fungal infections in body folds, such as under the breasts, where moisture and heat allow fungi to grow. To combat these problems, you may need to use more potent antiperspirants and wear cotton clothing next to the skin to absorb moisture. At menopause, dryness in the skin becomes a problem for many women, so wash your skin less frequently, and use moisturizers more often.

Age-Defying Solutions

You've been looking at the same face in the mirror every day of your life, then one day you notice a new brown growth here or an odd-looking mark there. You don't necessarily have to live with these age-related skin changes that are common to women of color. The answer may be no further than your drugstore or dermatologist's office. Some solutions to help you look like your (young) self again:

Problem: Uneven Skin Tone. This may manifest as blotchiness on the face or a stark contrast between facial skin and skin on the neck and chest. The primary cause is sun damage.

Solution. First, to prevent further discoloration and unevenness, use SPF 15 to 30 sunscreen generously on exposed skin every single day. Also wear sunhats and sun-protective clothing outdoors, and avoid direct sunlight. Talk to your dermatologist about applying a skin-bleaching cream containing 3 to 4 percent hydroquinone in addition to an exfoliating product such as glycolic acid cleanser or cream. In some cases, a series of glycolic acid or salicylic acid peels in your dermatologist's office may be the best option. By exfoliating dull skin and bleaching darkened areas, you will most likely be able to restore your natural tone. But this process takes time (at least several weeks or a few months) and it requires maintenance—routine sunscreen use and exfoliating with an at-home product.

Problem: New Growths. Brown or black growths, similar to moles, suddenly appear on the face (*dermatosis papulosa nigra*), neck (skin tags), or other parts of the body (*seborrheic keratoses*). The cause is unknown, though these benign growths do seem to run in families.

Solution. Talk to your dermatologist about having the growths removed. The physician can either snip off the growths surgically or apply an electric needle to the growth, causing it to burn and fall off. Either way, discomfort is minimal and the results are permanent, although new growths can develop at any time. (If you have ever developed keloid scars, however, you should not have any growths removed.)

Problem: Fine Lines and Wrinkles. This tends to be more of a concern for women of color with light skin, but all women of color may develop at least some wrinkles as they enter their forties, fifties, sixties, and beyond. Wrinkled skin is caused most likely by a combination of sun damage, slower collagen production, and years of facial expressions.

Solution: Over the years, skin researchers have come up with a number of different, very effective ways to try to eliminate or at least diminish wrinkles. The simplest way to make wrinkles less noticeable is through good skin care—use of moisturizers that make the skin look "plump" and sunscreen to prevent further wrinkles. To exfoliate dull, dry-looking skin and stimulate the production of new collagen, you might also consider using products or peels containing alphahydroxy acid (glycolic) or betahydroxy acid (salicylic). Products containing vitamin A are even more effective anti-aging agents, and come in over-the-counter (retinol) or prescription (Retin-A, Tazorac) formulas.

To target specific wrinkles such as those in the forehead or between the eyes, talk to a dermatologist about injections of Botox, a neurotoxin that paralyzes facial muscles in wrinkled areas. Another option is the use of filler substances, including collagen or fat, which are injected into lines and wrinkles. These treatments are effective but temporary.

For the most dramatic results, mature women may want to consider deeper chemical peels (Obagi), dermabrasion, or laser resurfacing, but these treatments are more likely to have adverse effects on skin of color. The most invasive and long-lasting wrinkle solution is cosmetic surgery, such as a partial or complete face-lift. However, any surgery carries risks and is expensive. (See chapter 5 for complete descriptions of cosmetic surgical techniques.)

What Are Those Red Spots on My Skin?

Some women of color will notice red spots or growths on the skin as they age. These growths, which vary in size from a pinpoint to the diameter of a pencil eraser, are known as *cherry angiomas*. While benign, the angiomas may be unsightly and, like other growths, increase in number as we age. You can ask a dermatologist to remove the growth through cauterization (burning with an electric needle). The procedure involves minimal pain and time.

Makeup Tips for Mature Women of Color

Because the nature of your skin is changing, your makeup routine should change as well. The makeup you wore at twenty, thirty, or forty won't necessarily complement your skin in later years. This is a time to experiment to find the shades and colors that look best on you. Don't hesitate to consult a makeup artist at a cosmetics counter if you need guidance. Here's how to stay looking forever young:

- Reconsider your skin type. It is likely to be more dry, so if you once had oily skin it may now actually be more like combination skin or normal skin type; previously normal skin may now be dry.
- Reconsider your skin tone. Owing to years of sun exposure, your facial skin may be noticeably darker than in previous years. If your skin tone has changed, your makeup shades will also need to change.
- Use concealer to camouflage uneven skin tone, which is more common in older skin of color. First, you'll need to select a concealer shade that is lighter than your current skin tone. It will also need to be formulated for your current skin type. You'll need more than one concealer because your skin type will likely change from season to season. Where discolorations are prominent, apply a concealer and blend.
- Make sure your foundation truly matches your skin tone. Test the shade by applying it to your entire face and viewing it with a mirror in natural light. If it is too light, keep looking and settle on a shade that more closely approximates your current tone. Steer clear of shades with undertones that are too orange or red. Once you've found the right shade, make sure it is a moisturizing liquid or cream foundation; avoid matte formulas, which can further dry skin. Apply one layer with a light touch evenly to skin with a makeup sponge.

- Blend foundation onto your neck to avoid a makeup line between the face and neck.

- Set your foundation with powder. A moisturizing loose powder or pressed powder will keep the skin from looking dry. Translucent powder will do for many women, but a pigmented shade that matches your foundation can further help camouflage uneven pigmentation. However, do not apply more than one light dusting of powder because too much powder will settle into—and emphasize—any fine lines or wrinkles.

- Apply blush below your cheekbones. For mature women, less may be more.

- Use an eyebrow pencil or shadow to add definition to brows that have been thinned through years of plucking. Light strokes between eyebrow hairs will look more natural than a straight line. Experiment with new eye shadow shades to complement your skin tone and blend, blend, blend. If you apply eyeliner and mascara, use a light hand. Dark eyeliner on the lower lid tends to emphasize under-eye circles, which may be more prominent now. If your eyelashes have thinned, consider using false ones instead of overdoing the mascara.

- Finish your face with moisturizing lipstick or lip gloss. Use matching lip liner around the edges of the lips first if your lip shape has become irregular. Also, if your lips have become drier, apply a lip balm containing SPF 15 sunscreen before your lipstick or gloss. As with foundation, blush, and eye shadows, experiment with colors—from soft beige or rose to burgundy or mocha—to find shades that best flatter you.

- Remove makeup daily with a makeup remover formulated for dry skin.

- Replace makeup frequently—every six months or so—since you are using moisturizing or oil-based formulas (foundation, powder) that can go bad more quickly. Eye makeup should be replaced every three months.

HAIR CARE AFTER FIFTY

When it comes to hair, mature women of color may experience some major challenges for the first time. One is increased dryness, owing primarily to estrogen loss. Another concern is thinning hair. Women of color tend to gray more gradually than White women, but at least some gray hairs will definitely emerge and increase in number, although often thin, gray, and silver hair tends to be more rough and dry than your other tresses. In addition to these natural changes, older women of color may notice other problems that have accumulated over time owing to harsh styling and cultural practices. These include permanent hair loss in the form of a receding hairline or lost volume, as well as split ends and breakage.

You *must* treat your hair especially gently now. If you've experienced significant hair loss, you may want to consider changing your hair styling regimen completely. (See chapter 14 if you have alopecia.) Many older women opt for shorter styles or naturals, which are easier to maintain. If you relax your hair, do it on a less frequent schedule—no more than four times a year. Whatever style you choose, be sure to wash weekly and condition with a deep penetrating or restructuring conditioner. Weekly hot-oil treatments will also combat dry, brittle, and dull-looking hair. If you can air-dry or wrap your hair and still maintain your style, do so to avoid the heat of hair dryers.

Only if your hair is in relatively good condition, consider covering gray with a semi-permanent professional dye or rinse. Choose a shade only slightly lighter than your natural hair color for a subtle effect. Remember that color-treated hair will be dryer, so keep using conditioners and hot-oil treatments regularly. Because your hair is more fragile, permanent hair coloring should be done less frequently—perhaps only twice a year—but a hair rinse can be used more frequently.

HELP FOR AGING HANDS

When women of color worry about their age and appearance, they are most often concerned about how their face and hair look. But because our hands are just as vulnerable to the sun and other elements, they can also show signs of maturity, including dryness, skin thinning, and, in lighter skinned women, even age spots. To keep your hands looking youthful, don't neglect them. Take these steps:

- Apply SPF 15 to 30 sunscreen generously to your hands as well as your face, every single day.
- Use a rich moisturizer on your hands each day, and reapply as often as needed. Ones to try are Neutrogena Hand Cream and Amlactin Lotion.
- Select moisturizers containing exfoliating agents such as glycolic acid or retinol to remove dry, dull skin.
- Avoid harsh soaps.
- Wear cotton gloves under plastic or rubber gloves for any wet housework.
- Consult a dermatologist if you develop age spots. Often they can be treated with hydroquinone bleaching creams.

Maintaining Youthful Nails

Nails become particularly dry as we age. Splitting and breaking of the nails are common complaints among mature women of color. The following tips will help keep your nails strong and beautiful:

- Minimize contact with water by wearing cotton gloves covered by rubber gloves while doing wet work.
- Moisturize the nails three or four time per day with a rich moisturizer.
- File nails gently and straight across (avoid an oval-shaped nail).
- Do not use your nails as an implement.
- Apply a coat of clear nail polish weekly.

CHAPTER 14

HAIR-RAISING SOLUTIONS

Too much hair in certain areas and not enough hair in others—these hair issues have become the number one problem for many Black women. You may have assumed that hair loss mainly affects men and a few unlucky older women. However, hair loss in Brown women is epidemic and it can appear in women at any age. *Alopecia* is the technical term for hair loss. It may take several forms. The first form of alopecia is thinning of the density of the hair. If this occurs, you may be able actually to see the scalp through the hair or you may have noticed that a part in your hair is wider than before. Alopecia may also take the form of the complete absence of hair in small or larger patches on the scalp (areas where the scalp is "clean"). Finally, alopecia may appear as breakage of the strands of hair, resulting in hair of multiple lengths with very short sections in some areas.

A number of factors, including illness, hormonal shifts, certain medications, and particularly harsh hair-styling practices, can contribute to hair thinning or loss. Whatever the cause, if hair loss occurs, it can be alarming and devastating to your appearance and your self-esteem.

Black women are particularly susceptible to alopecia because of common cultural styling practices that are harmful to the hair and scalp. Whether you wear your hair relaxed or natural, you've probably exposed it to some damaging styling techniques at some time or even regularly. Chemical relaxers, hot combs, hot dryers, tight braids, heavy weaves, long heavy locks, taut ponytails, tight rollers, and even vigorous combing all can lead to weakened hair strands and injured hair follicles. In addition, researchers have found that, for reasons that are not entirely understood, the hair follicles in Black women may not be as well anchored to the scalp as the follicles of Whites. The combination of more vulnerable follicles and more destructive hair-care habits creates the risk of a pervasive hair-loss problem for women of African descent.

But hair loss is not inevitable. The major cause of alopecia in women of color—hair-care practices combined with harsh styling—can be prevented, and in some cases, hair loss can be halted and even reversed. Many women do not realize that over time their hair (like the rest of their body) changes, so styles and processes that were once well tolerated by your hair may now cause damage. Other types of alopecia can also be addressed through a variety of hair-loss treatments as well strategies to camouflage thinning hair and bald spots.

If you've experienced hair thinning or loss, don't ignore it—it probably will not just go away. Because alopecia can be the sign of an underlying medical problem, you should see a dermatologist to get the problem diagnosed and properly treated. Hair loss can be most effectively addressed when it is caught early, so consult a dermatologist sooner rather than later. Many of my patients come in much too late—that is, when the hair loss is in an advanced, final stage. Either the stimulation of new growth or cessation of further hair loss may have been possible if these patients had just come in earlier.

The other hair-related problem that plagues many a woman of color is excess hair growth, whether it appears on the face or on other parts of the body. (Sometimes excessive hair growth is a sign of a hormonal imbalance and you should consult your doctor.) You are probably aware of the variety of hair removal methods, from waxing to the new Vaniqa cream. However, you may not know all the risks associated with techniques such as laser hair removal or the potential for pigmentary problems if the skin is injured. This chapter outlines the pros and cons of each technique and provides a chart to help you pick the best—and safest—solution.

The Roots of Hair Loss

Alopecia may be triggered by several different factors, including:

- Chemical relaxers that are not used as directed and/or combined with permanent hair dyes or other chemical processes.
- Hair pulling from braids, weaves, tight ponytails, hair rollers
- Hair pulling from natural styles such as long heavy locks or very tight twists
- High heat from blow dryers, hot combs, curling irons, or electric rollers
- Hormonal fluctuations (during the postpartum period or with the discontinuation of oral contraceptive pills)
- Hormonal abnormalities (polycystic ovarian syndrome or PCOS, adrenal disease)
- Hypothyroidism or hyperthyroidism
- Chronic illness (e.g, lupus, HIV/AIDS)
- Severe iron-deficiency anemia
- Fungal infection/ringworm
- Bacterial infections (folliculitis)
- Severe fever or infection
- Surgery
- Low-protein diet
- Sudden, dramatic weight change
- Certain medications
- Chemotherapy
- Extreme stress

Quiz: *Are You Harming Your Hair?*

Women of color too often assume that our hair styling practices are benign, and that our hair can take a battery of heat, chemicals, pulling, and tugging and continue to grow and look healthy. But as a dermatologist and a Black woman, I know this is all too often not the case. We also forget that our hair is ever changing and what it was able to once tolerate, may now cause severe damage and loss. Take this quiz to assess your hair care "intelligence quotient."

1. How often do you relax your hair (including touch-ups)?
    a. Eight or more times a year
    b. Six times a year
    c. Four times a year or less
    d. I don't relax my hair

2. When your hair is being relaxed, you have the stylist wash out the relaxer when the scalp feels:
    a. like it's burning
    b. like it's tingling severely and you can't take it anymore
    c. like it's tingling slightly
    d. I don't relax my hair

3. When you have your hair cornrowed or braided, how does your scalp feel?
    a. I have a headache for days afterward and I am unable to move or wrinkle my forehead for a few days
    b. It feels uncomfortably tight for a few hours or days
    c. It feels fine (no tightness or pulling)
    d. I don't braid my hair

4. To style your hair straight, you or your stylist:
    a. use a handheld blow dryer followed by a curling iron
    b. use a handheld blow dryer and pull the hair straighter with a comb or brush
    c. use a hooded dryer with rollers or a wrap
    d. I gently smooth my hair back into a ponytail and air-dry

5. When you add a weave to your hair, it:

    a. falls past the shoulders and adds noticeable weight to the hair

    b. is bonded (glued) to your scalp

    c. is light and/or falls to shoulder length or shorter

    d. I don't use weaves

6. When you pull your hair back into a ponytail(s), the skin at your hairline:

    a. feels tight and appears pulled

    b. feels a little tight

    c. feels comfortable

    d. I gently smooth my hair into a loose ponytail

7. Your locks are

    a. long, thick, and heavy

    b. halfway down your back or past your shoulders

    c. relatively short or ear length, thin to medium diameter, and of uniform size

    d. I don't wear locks

Analysis:

You've probably figured out that if your answers were mostly *d*s, you're not treating your hair very harshly and your hair care IQ is high. If you checked mostly *c*s, you're probably styling your hair responsibly. Mostly *a* and *b* answers are an indication that your hair-styling habits are harmful to your hair and scalp, and may someday lead to damage and hair thinning, if not hair loss. To improve your hair-care IQ, see chapter 4 for advice on styling your hair the way you like without destroying it in the process. Remember that pain and discomfort—whether from chemicals, heat, or pulling the hair—are *not* normal! It's worth it to learn to treat your hair and scalp more gently.

WHAT WOMEN OF COLOR MUST KNOW ABOUT HAIR LOSS

All of us shed some hair routinely as part of the hair's normal growth cycle. In fact, it's normal to loose up to one hundred hairs per day. At any given time approximately 90 percent of the hair on our heads is actively growing (known as the anagen phase); the other 8 percent is in a resting or dormant state (catagen phase). After a few months, the remaining 2 percent of the resting hair sheds (telogen phase), resulting in a loss that is not noticeable. The shed hair is replaced when the cycle starts all over again.

However, hair loss, or alopecia, occurs when this growth cycle is disrupted, either when clumps of hair fall out from the roots, hair breaks off at or near the scalp, or it ceases to grow altogether. There are a number of reasons this might happen.

Sometimes hair loss is a normal consequence of life stages, such as during the postpartum period when hormonal changes cause large amounts of hair to fall out (termed *telogen effluvium*), or during menopause, when a lack of hormones may make hair thinner. At other times, hair loss is a short-term response to a health problem—a sudden weight loss, severe infection or illness, and even stress. After the crisis, hair usually resumes its normal growth.

Too frequently for Black women, though, hair thinning or loss is progressive and permanent. It's due to years of very harsh styling practices that damage either hair strands or hair follicles. The three main types of hair loss that afflict Black women are traction alopecia, follicular degeneration syndrome, and hair breakage. But there are other types you should be aware of as well.

Your Hair-Loss Evaluation

When evaluating your hair loss, your doctor may perform some or all of the following tests:

- Blood tests: thyroid function tests (TSH, T_4), hormonal evaluation (DHEA-sulfate, free testosterone level, total testosterone level), lupus tests (ANA), test for anemia (CBC), test for syphilis (RPR)
- Scalp biopsy (H & E and immunofluorescence)
- Cultures (fungal and/or bacterial)

Hair Scare: How Much Loss Is Too Much?

You may sometimes wonder if the amount of hair that you shed when you wash or style it is normal. The human head normally sheds between fifty and hundred hairs per day. You'll know that hair loss is abnormal if:

- It sheds more than a hundred hairs within a twenty-four-hour period.
- You notice clumps of hair in the shower, or in your brush or comb.
- You wake up to find more hair than usual on your pillow.

Examine the shed hairs to determine if there are small white balls on the ends of the hair (sign of a telogen hair). Also take a close look at the hair near your scalp. Are there a number of strands that have only grown out to an inch or so? Is the hair along your hairline thin or broken off? Is the scalp discolored or is there a rash or bumps? When in doubt, schedule an appointment with a dermatologist for a complete evaluation. Hold off on any touch-ups or hair treatments until you've identified the source of the problem. And remember, your hairdresser or stylist, although knowledgeable about your hair, is not a substitute for a dermatologist who is well trained in Black hair health.

Types of Alopecia and Treatment

The Condition: Traction Alopecia. Pulling the hair very tightly into braids, ponytails, or rollers causes this form of hair loss. Another source of this problem is the weight of braids or weaves with long extension and locks. When you pull too hard, hair strands can break and even come right out of your scalp. More important, the hair root or follicle will become inflamed from the chronic pulling or traction, and small bumps will develop (you may have noticed that your daughter has plait bumps). The inflammation will then lead to destruction of the hair follicle and permanent loss of hair. Over time, bald spots can develop, particularly along the hairline and the area above the ears. We have all seen women whose hairline now begins in the middle of their scalp. Since the hair loss happens gradually, you may not even notice it until the bald spot develops or your hairline recedes significantly.

The Treatment. It may seem obvious, but it's time to stop pulling your hair out. To save your hair, you may need to switch hairstyles altogether. However, if your hair loss is minimal and you want to continue to braid your hair or plait your child's hair, for instance, you can make adjustments, such as wearing looser braids, plaiting the hair loosely, and wearing shorter weaves or locks. Women of color often pull tightly on hair to make it look smooth or straighter in a ponytail or bun. A better solution might be to apply a hair gel or a dab of conditioner to the hair to help it to lie flatter and straighter. More manageable hair will look smooth and neat without all that pulling, so wash and deep-condition regularly. To camouflage bald spots or a receding hairline you might consider brushing your hair toward the hairline or coloring the scalp with a scalp pencil. You can find scalp pencils at a local beauty supply store; apply as you would an eyebrow pencil, with short strokes in the direction of hair growth.

The Condition: Follicular Degeneration Syndrome (a type of scarring alopecia). This form of hair loss is poorly understood, but is most likely caused by repeated and frequent but unnoticed damage to the hair follicles. In Black women we suspect this damage is due to the combination of our various hair-care practices. These factors may include hot-combing (with microscopic drops of hot hair oil dripping onto and damaging the hair follicles); chemical relaxing (the severe tingling and burning that occurs when the application directions are not followed most likely produces inflammation and destruction of the hair follicles); tight rollers or curlers used to set the hair (with chronic pulling or traction); and blow-drying (with excessive heat applied to the scalp and hot oil droplets destroying the follicles). Once the hair follicles become damaged or destroyed, scar tissue results and hair *will never regrow*.

The Treatment. Since dermatologists do not know the exact cause of follicular degeneration syndrome, outlining a treatment is difficult. We think that the first step is to stop any styling practice that may be causing or contributing to the hair loss. That means no hot combs, no tightly applied rollers or braids, blow-drying, or relaxers for a period of at least six to nine months. This will allow your hair follicles and hair an opportunity to repair themselves. Your dermatologist can help you determine when—and if—you can resume styling. If the hair follicles have not been damaged beyond repair, you may, for example, be able to resume your hair-care practices but with modifications. For example, you can switch from hot combs and blow dryers to hooded dryers or wraps to prevent future damage. Taking a break from harsh styling and substituting gentler techniques often allow the inflammation to resolve, the scalp to heal, and hair growth to resume. However, your dermatologist may prescribe cortisone to be applied to the scalp to treat any residual inflammation.

The Condition: Hair Breakage. Hair breakage may be due to a variety of factors that damage the strands of hair. The breakage may occur repeatedly in a certain area of the scalp, and this area varies from individual to individual. You might call it the weak area of your scalp. Often the hair feels dry and brittle in the area of breakage. Excessive heat, dyes, and chemicals are common precipitating factors to hair breakage. Breakage is more common when multiple processes are applied to the hair. Trichotillomania (see box, page 260) is another cause of breakage. In either case, the hair is of varying lengths.

The Treatment. The first step is to give your hair a break (no pun intended) or rest so that it can repair itself and become healthy again. Consider washing and conditioning weekly and eliminating the heat, dyes, and relaxers for a minimum of three months. Hot-oil treatments or overnight oil treatments may also help to restore the original suppleness of the hair. During this reparative time, wearing a wig or the hair pulled back loosely is an alternative.

The Condition: Alopecia Areata. People who have this type of alopecia develop small dime- or quarter-sized round bald spots on the scalp or other hair-bearing area of the body. The area of involvement is totally "clean"—that is, devoid of hair—and the scalp has a smooth appearance. Hair tends to shed in patches for a few months, then may regrow for no apparent reason. A pattern of loss and regrowth can continue unpredictably for years, or go into remission. In a few individuals, the hair loss may involve the entire scalp (*alopecia totalis*). The cause of *alopecia areata* is not known but it probably involves an immune system abnormality. Hair loss may be accompanied by thickened, brittle nails, thyroid problems, vitiligo, or anemia.

The Treatment. Consult a dermatologist, who will prescribe one of the following treatments: corticosteroid creams, solutions, or injections; or oral medication such as cortisone pill or other topical medications (Anthralin, Rogaine). The success of alopecia areata treatment varies, and you may need to experiment with different treatments to find out what works for you.

The Condition: Androgenic Alopecia. This form of hair thinning is generally hereditary. It's characterized by thinning in the crown area extending toward the hairline. The hair in the back of the scalp (occiput) often remains fuller and thicker. You may have noticed that the part in your hair is becoming wider and you are able to see your scalp through the thinning hair. Unlike men, you will not become completely bald. However, the hair can continue to thin slowly over time. The underlying scalp appears normal.

The Treatment. Medications such as Rogaine (there are varieties for men and women) may help improve the condition. Talk to your dermatologist about additional therapies such as hair transplantation. To camouflage thinned areas, you might also use hair dyes to color the scalp or a wig. Loose weaves are also a good solution.

The Condition: Telogen Effluvium. The most common cause of this temporary hair loss is the drop in hormones during the postpartum period or the discontinuation of oral contraceptive pills. Hair loss may be significant, and very frightening, with handfuls of hair coming out at a time. The hair loss occurs diffusely all over the scalp. A clue to telogen effluvium is the presence of small white balls on the ends of the hair (telogen hairs). However, normal hair growth typically resumes on its own since telogen effluvium is a self-limiting problem. Other causes of telogen effluvium include illness (especially those with high fever), surgery, dramatic weight change (especially if associated with caloric or protein deprivation), and psychological stress, which all disrupt the hair's normal growth pattern.

The Treatment. Since the causes of telogen effluvium are typically short term, the hair loss is usually not permanent. It is important to treat the hair gently and to not overmanipulate it. Minimize brushing and combing and hold off on touchups. If the hair doesn't grow back, see your dermatologist to rule out another problem.

The Condition: Drug-Induced Alopecia. A number of different medications can disrupt normal hair growth pattern and cause hair loss. This hair loss is usually diffuse, affecting all areas of the scalp. The offending agents include drugs taken for medical problems such as high blood pressure, high cholesterol, heart disease, arthritis, and depression, among others. (See "Is Your Medication Causing Your Hair Loss?" page 258).

The Treatment. Talk to your physician to make sure the medication is the source of your hair loss. Your doctor should be able to help you select a substitute medication of another class that will not cause hair loss.

Is Your Medication Causing Your Hair Loss?

The following drugs might contribute to hair loss:

Coumadin (an anticoagulant or blood thinner)

Atenolol (a beta blocker)

Lithium (an antiseizure medication)

Valproic acid (an antiseizure medication)

Vitamin A excess

Chemotherapy

The Condition: Scarring Alopecia. This form of alopecia is specific to diseases, such as *discoid lupus erythematosus* (DLE), *lichen planopilaris* (LPP), *pseudopelade of brocq*, and *follicular degeneration syndrome* (see above), that scar the hair follicles. Once the hair follicles are scarred they cannot produce hair. You will notice discolorations (light, dark, or even pink) on the scalp and various types of rashes or bumps with many of the scarring alopecias. Hair loss in this case may be permanent.

The Treatment. Your physician will probably prescribe corticosteroids to reduce the inflammation that contributes to scarring. If all of the follicles have not been destroyed already, some other medications may be helpful. Sun protection is also important for discoid lupus.

The Condition: *Tinea Capitus* (fungal infections) and *Bacterial Folliculitis* (bacterial infection). Women with either of these problems may notice red bumps, pus bumps, and significant scaling of the scalp. Hair loss in patches is another noticeable feature. The scalp may be very itchy and inflamed.

The Treatment. You must see the dermatologist for prescription medication to treat either the fungal or bacterial infection. The antifungal medication will need to be administered for as long as six or eight weeks. Seek treatment immediately, since further hair loss may occur.

The Condition: Traumatic Alopecia. Many women do not realize that they can do severe damage to their remaining hair follicles by gluing weaves onto their scalp. When they remove the weave, precious hair comes out as well.

The Treatment. Never allow a stylist to use hair bonding or glue to attach your weave. Although there are products that dissolve the glue, you will still pull some hair out when removing a weave attached in this manner. Ask the stylist to loosely weave hair in instead.

The Condition: Syphilis-Induced Alopecia. Diseases that you might not think of can also produce hair loss. For example, hair loss may be the only manifestation of the secondary form of syphilis. With this disease, the hair loss is patchy and has a "moth-eaten" appearance. Alternatively, it may just appear as diffuse thinning.

The Treatment. Treatment with the appropriate antibiotics will result in the regrowth of hair.

Cancer and Hair Loss

Because African Americans and Hispanics have higher rates of many different forms of cancer, hair loss owing to cancer treatment is a particular concern for us. While killing cancer cells in the body, chemotherapy treatments also harm healthy cells, including the cells in your hair. That's why cancer patients lose much of their hair during treatment. Hair growth usually returns to normal after treatment, but in the meantime, patients can disguise the loss with wigs, colorful scarves and head wraps, and hats. (The Breast Cancer Resource Center of Princeton YWCA offers free wigs to women nationwide who need financial assistance at www.bcrcnj.org. Cancer Care also offers free wigs. For more

hair-loss help, see the National Alliance of Breast Cancer Organization's website, www.nabco.org.)

What Is Trichotillomania?

Some women of color pull on the hair on their head, in their eyebrows, and even their eyelashes until the hairs fall out. This psychological disturbance is known as *trichotillomania*. Like nail biting, hair pulling is often a coping mechanism for dealing with stress. Besides the fact that the pulling is painful, it can also lead to permanent hair loss. If you have a tendency to twist and pull your hair when you feel nervous or pressured, talk to your doctor. You may be suffering from an anxiety disorder that can be treated with stress-reducing activities, therapy, or medication.

Rx: Hair Reconstruction Regimen

If your hair is dry, brittle, and breaking, the following regimen, including products, will help to repair it (also see the websites www.drsusantaylor.net and www.society-hilldermatology.com):

- Discontinue relaxers, texturizers, and permanent hair dyes for a six- to nine-month period.
- Trim the dead ends, and if it applies to you, even the length of your hair to one length all over the scalp.
- While the hair is being repaired, pull your hair back gently into a ponytail or consider wearing a wig when you leave your home.
- Discontinue the application of excessive heat to your hair. That means avoidance of blow dryers, hot combs, and curling irons.

In addition, institute a hair reconstruction regimen such as the following (see also the websites listed above):

1. Each Friday night, saturate the hair and scalp with the hair reconstruction oil. Cover with a clear shower cap, which remains in place overnight. Before removing the cap, apply a warm towel over the cap for ten minutes or sit under a hood dryer for ten minutes.

2. Remove the cap and wash the hair thoroughly with the oil-removing shampoo and rinse.

3. Lather up with the conditioning shampoo and leave it for two minutes.

4. Rinse thoroughly and then apply the deep conditioner for fifteen minutes. You may consider sitting under a hooded dryer during this time or wrap a warm towel around your head.

5. Rinse, comb with a wide-tooth comb, and gently dry the hair (either air-dry or sit under a hooded dryer).

6. Throughout the week, apply the hair repair cream to the ends of the hair.

7. For itching and flaking of the scalp, throughout the week apply a small amount of the hair reconstruction oil directly onto the scalp.

8. While sleeping, wear a satin scarf or cap so that the hair does not get caught on the pillowcase and break.

Strict adherence to this regime for the next six to nine months will result in healthier, softer, and stronger hair.

HAIR REMOVAL

Clearing your skin of unwanted, excess hair is as simple as whipping out your razor or making a trip to the beauty salon, right? Not so fast! For women of color with curly hair on the face, neck, underarms, or legs, hair removal carries the risk of ingrown hairs, which irritate and inflame the skin. This condition, known as *pseudofolliculitis barbae* (PFB), is more common in Black men (see chapter 15), but afflicts women as well. Affected skin can become bumpy and discolored. In addition, if you don't remove hair carefully, you can develop small nicks or cuts, which can also lead to hyperpigmentation and even keloids. Black women who are prone to hyperpigmentation should be especially cautious about removing unwanted hair. Those with keloidal scars should consult a dermatologist about how to clear the skin of hair safely.

Excess Hair and Your Health

Often excessive hair growth is hereditary and your mother, aunts, and sisters will also have excessive hair. However, at other times it indicates a medical problem. For example, if you have too much hair on your face in addition to having irregular periods and severe acne, you may have a condition called *polycystic ovarian syndrome* (PCOS). Some women with PCOS also develop dark, velvety skin on the neck, breasts, and inner thighs, known as *acanthosis nigricans*. If your excess hair growth is accompanied by other symptoms such as irregular or absent periods, see your doctor. Another cause of excess hair growth is hyperthyroidism, or overactive thyroid. Some women who have multiple sclerosis or who have suffered from anorexia nervosa may develop excessive hair growth. Finally, after a head injury, excessive hair growth may develop.

Medications and Excess Hair

Some medications may be the cause of your excessive hair growth. Discuss the possibility with your physician to see if another medication can be substituted. Some of the troublesome medications are:

Diazoxide (for hypertension)

Phenytoin (for seizures)

Cyclosporin (to prevent transplantation rejections)

Streptomycin (an antibiotic)

Acetazolamide (for glaucoma)

How to Get Smooth, Hairless Skin—Safely

The hair removal method you choose will depend on many factors, including the amount of hair, its texture and location, and your preference for regrowth time. Common methods include:

Plucking. A mildly painful method most commonly applied to the eyebrow area and upper lip. Too much plucking can lead to thinned eyebrows, so be sure to only remove stray hairs. Plucking hair in the chin area or on the neck can lead to worsening of *pseudofolliculitis barbae* (razor bumps) and it is not a recommended method of hair removal in these areas. As the hair is plucked, it breaks below the surface of the skin and pierces the hair follicle, causing damage and inflammation beneath the surface of the skin.

Shaving. A quick method typically applied to the legs and underarms. Because it cuts hair at the skin surface, this method is most likely to result in irritated skin and ingrown hairs. If you choose to shave, always use a fresh razor on clean skin moistened with water and soap, or a shaving cream or gel. Shave gently in the direction of hair growth to avoid ingrown hairs. Never shave your face.

Cutting. The best method for those occasional hairs that grow on your nipples, chin, or from a mole. Cut the hair with a mustache scissors or a small pair of scissors. This is preferable to plucking hairs in these delicate areas.

Depilatory (hair removal creams). This method is best for small areas that are not too easily irritated, such as the upper lip, chin, and bikini area. Depilatories, however, contain chemicals that may be harsh on the skin and this often leads to irritation of the skin and redness. Use the product as directed and be sure to test it first. If irritation develops at any time, discontinue use.

Waxing. This method stings but it's quick and keeps you hair-free for weeks at a time. Wax is usually applied in a salon to the upper lip, underarm, bikini line, or legs. At-home kits can be messy and not as effective. Whether in the salon or at home, be careful not to burn the skin with the hot wax.

Sugaring. Also done in salons, this method uses a sugar and lemon mixture to remove hair from the roots. Though less painful than waxing, it may cause irritation.

Electrolysis. This method involves the use of an electric current to destroy hair follicles. A needle is inserted into the hair follicle and a current destroys the hair and follicle. It takes time—often repeat visits over months or years—and is more expensive than most methods. Although electrolysis has the advantage of giving long-term results, it causes redness initially and can scar the skin.

Laser Hair Removal. Laser hair removal targets the hair follicle with a beam of light that heats and destroys the hair. Since a large area can be done, it requires far fewer visits than electrolysis. Results are long-term, although it is possible for some hair to regrow. However, this method can remove pigment from skin of color or cause dark areas on the skin. It is also critically important that the hair removal laser be performed by a dermatologist knowledgeable about skin of color. The Long Pulse Diode and Alexandrite Lasers are preferable for skin of color because they have a less harmful effect on the skin. Note: Because lasers can cause severe damage to skin if applied by unskilled hands, be sure to only get treatment from a board-certified dermatologist or health-care professional.

Prescription Cream (Vaniqa). One of the newest hair removal methods, Vaniqa retards hair growth at the root level by blocking a hormone that causes hair to grow. Vaniqa is helpful in about 58 percent of women who use it. Although it is generally well tolerated, in some women it can cause irritation and bumps.

HAIR REMOVAL CHART

METHOD	WHERE TO DO IT	BODY PART(S)	BENEFITS	RISKS
Plucking	At home/salon	Eyebrow, lip	Simple, precise Lasts a week or more	Mild pain
Shaving	At home	Underarms, legs	Simple, fast Lasts days	Irritation, ingrown hairs, hyperpigmentation
Depilatory	At home	Lip, chin, bikini, underarms, legs	Simple, fast Lasts a week or more	Irritation, messy
Waxing	At home/salon	Lip, brow, chin, underarms, bikini, legs	Fast Lasts several weeks	Irritation, pain, ingrown hairs
Sugaring	At home/salon	Lip, brow, chin, underarms, bikini, legs	Fast Lasts several weeks	Irritation, pain
Electrolysis	Salon/office	Lip, brow, chin, underarms, bikini, legs	Long-term, sometimes permanent results	Pain, scarring, hyperpigmentation, repeated regrowth
Lasers	Salon/derm. office	Lip, brow, chin, underarms, bikini, legs	Long-term, often permanent results	Irritation, burning, hyperpigmentation or hypopigmentation
Vaniqa	Prescription	Lip, chin, underarms, legs	Long-term results	Irritation, bumps

CHAPTER 15

JUST FOR HIM

Like women of color, men of color enjoy the benefits of having skin that gives them a warmer complexion, greater natural sun protection, and fewer signs of aging as compared to White men. Also like women of color, their hair tends to be more curly and coarse, or thick. However, men of color tend to suffer from some of the downsides as well: pigmentation problems in the skin and hair that is prone to growing into the skin after it's been shaved or cut.

Men of color are particularly susceptible to two common skin conditions: *pseudofolliculitis barbae* (PFB), commonly known as razor bumps, and *acne keloidalis nuchae* (AKN), a problem characterized by bumps and keloids that develop at the nape of the neck after hair cutting. Needless to say, the bumps and scars caused by these conditions are irritating and unsightly. In most cases, razor bumps cause hyperpigmentation, or skin darkening, and the bumps can even become infected or cause keloids. Generally, the two conditions are uncomfortable, embarrassing, and a source of frustration for men who try to get rid of them.

To avoid these problems and keep their skin, hair, and nails looking great, men of color don't necessarily need to follow time-consuming grooming regimens, but they should adopt good skin and hair-care practices. Nail care matters as well, particularly for professional men. As men of color learn how to shave and attend to their skin properly, they'll need to teach their sons these skills as well.

PSEUDOFOLLICULITIS BARBAE (PFB)

Both Black and Hispanic men and women are affected by ingrown hairs (PFB) and the consequent formation of bumps and hyperpigmentation. However, PFB is more common in Black and Hispanic men—particularly those who shave. It has been estimated that between 45 and 75 percent of Black men in the military have experienced PFB.

Men of all races and ethnic backgrounds shave, so why are Black and Hispanic men more prone to bumps? The hair follicles of these men (and women, too) are curved and the hair tends to be curly or coiled. As hairs emerge from the curved follicles, they grow almost parallel to the skin surface instead of away from the skin. While shaving, the cut hair develops a sharply pointed end, and it is this pointed end that curves and punctures the skin, growing inward. This ingrowing hair causes an inflammatory reaction in the skin, irritation, and unsightly bumps, technically known as *pseudofolliculitis barbae*. Many women of color tweeze or pluck their facial hair. With this form of hair removal, the hair breaks below the surface of the skin, pierces the hair follicle, and then produces the same inflammatory response and bumps.

The bumps may be small or large, and sometimes they cover a large area of skin. Commonly, the cheeks, chin, neck, and submental (the area under the chin) areas are affected. As is the case with all people of color, irritated skin can easily become hyperpigmented or darkened unevenly. That's why the jawline and necks of many men of color are rough, bumpy, and darker than the rest of their skin.

To avoid persistent razor bumps, some men of color simply choose to grow beards and never shave. But when this is not desirable or feasible for the work environment, men can learn more skin-friendly ways to remove facial hair.

How Often Should You Shave?

The frequency of shaving will affect PFB. I recommend shaving every day instead of twice a week, which is the common practice of many

Black and Hispanic men. By shaving daily, many of the hairs do not grow long enough to pierce the skin. If you switch over to shaving every day, the first two weeks may be difficult and you may experience transient irritation. Be sure to use an over-the-counter hydrocortisone cream for that two-week period to decrease any potential irritation.

Skin-friendly Shaving Method

How to do it:

1. Gently cleanse your face and neck with a mild cleanser. Leave skin damp.
2. Apply a shaving cream or gel (such as Nivea Shaving Cream, Edge Shaving Gel, or Neutrogena Skin Clearing Shave Cream) to your mustache, beard, and/or sideburns. Leave it on for a few minutes to completely soften the hairs.
3. Use a single-edge razor (double and triple blade razors worsen PFB) of the disposable variety, or even better, a bump-fighting razor, available at drugstores.
4. Shave with the razor in the direction of the hair growth, not against the grain.
5. Rinse the razor free of hair and cream between strokes.
6. Shave each area of skin only once. Do not stretch the skin to get a closer shave since this will worsen PFB.
7. Rinse the face with lukewarm water and pat dry.
8. After shaving, instead of applying a potentially irritating after-shave, try a lotion containing an alphahydroxy acid such as MD Forte or Alpha Hydrox (which has been demonstrated to improve PFB). This will soothe just-shaven skin and gently exfoliate it at the same time.

To prevent ingrown hairs, carefully check your beard between shaves. To loosen and dislodge hairs that start to grow inward, gently rub skin in the opposite direction of hair growth with a clean washcloth or a soft baby toothbrush. You might want to do this before you go to bed each night or before a shave. Try not to pluck ingrown hairs out. Instead, gently turn the curving hairs outward and then shave. If proper shaving and vigilance do not prevent ingrown hairs, or if bumps enlarge, turn the skin dark or become infected (itchy, painful), see a dermatologist for prescription medication or laser treatments. The sooner you seek care for PFB, the easier the problem will be to resolve. You'll also minimize any discoloration to your skin.

Alternatives to the Razor

To cope with persistent PFB, talk to your dermatologist about the following alternatives to shaving.

Depilatories. Over-the-counter hair removal creams will remove unwanted hair at the skin surface, avoiding the friction of razors. These products break the disulfide bonds that hold hairs in curled or coiled position, and the hair falls off at the surface of the skin. The results last longer—from a few days to a week—giving your skin a break between applications. A widely used product is Magic Shave Powder. However, the major disadvantage of depilatories is that they can cause skin burning, irritation, and redness. Often depilatories also have an unpleasant smell.

Hair Clippers. Many men cut beard hair with hair clippers. Although it does not afford a "close" shave, it maintains a hair length of approximately 1 mm (the length of a grain of rice). A hair that is 1 mm or longer will not pierce the skin's surface and the risk of PFB is minimized.

Electric Razors. Some men (but not all) can minimize their PFB through the use of an electric razor. Avoiding nicks and cuts with this type of razor is an advantage for some men.

Medicated Cream. Newer prescription creams, such as Vaniqa, are medicated to slow hair growth between shaves. Although this medication was designed and approved for blocking the growth of facial hair in women, many male patients also use it. This medication slows the growth process enough so that fewer ingrown hairs occur. You will still have to shave, but often for men the growth is less dense.

Electrolysis. This hair removal method is designed to stop hair growth permanently by destroying the follicle with an electrical pulse. Although it is a slow process that requires several repeat visits over many years in some cases, it is effective. However, electrolysis is slightly painful and can cause redness and scabbing, which can lead to skin discoloration and scarring in men of color.

Laser Hair Removal. The most recent form of permanent hair removal, this method retards hair growth by zapping the hair follicle with a beam of light. Laser hair removal removes hair more quickly than electrolysis, requiring between five and seven treatments over as many months. Although generally well tolerated, it has been known to cause burning or discolorations in the skin. It is also critically important that the laser hair removal be performed by dermatologists knowledgeable in brown skin. The Long Pulse Diode and Alexandrite Lasers are preferable for skin of color because they have a less harmful effect on the skin. Laser hair removal is not an option for men who want to be able to grow a full beard in the future.

Treatment of PFB

Although there is no cure for PFB, there are several safe and effective treatments that your dermatologist can prescribe. These include:

- Oral antibiotics: tetracycline, minocycline, and erythromycin
- Topical antibiotics: erythromycin or clindamycin, alone or combined with benzoyl peroxide
- Retinoids: adapalene, tretinoin, tazarotene
- Skin lighteners: 4 percent hydroquinone

ACNE KELOIDALIS NUCHAE (AKN)

Although dermatologists do not know the exact cause of *acne keloidalis nuchae* (AKN), we think that shaving the hair along the back of the neck poses additional hazards for men of color and the risk of developing AKN. This effort to achieve a neat, polished appearance is very irritating to the skin and may produce ingrown hairs, nicks and cuts in the skin. Irritation and dryness in the area make men want to scratch this area, which can cause the skin to become even more inflamed. Chronic rubbing from shirt collars may also irritate the skin. Over time, chronic inflammation and scratching can lead to bleeding, infection, and the formation of small firm bumps much like razor bumps on the face. In the worst cases, the bumps develop into large keloidal scars. This condition is known as *acne keloidalis nuchae* or *folliculitis keloidalis*. Whatever you call it, it's painful and difficult to treat.

Although AKN is most likely to occur on the back to the neck, it can develop on the scalp as well, in men who shave their heads with razors or otherwise irritate the scalp continuously with harsh combing or chemical treatments. Often it will develop even without significant overt irritation. However, once AKN has developed, it may trigger hair loss or bald spots. The combination of bumps and keloids on the scalp or neck is quite unsightly and can lead to great embarrassment and diminished self-esteem.

Prevention: Safe Scalp and Neck Care

To keep your scalp and posterior neck free of irritation and AKN:

- Wash your hair and neck gently once or twice a week.
- Try to avoid close haircuts and by all means avoid nicks and cuts to the area.
- Do not pick at any trapped hairs under the skin.
- If you must shave your hair, apply a shaving cream or gel and use only sharp,

clean single-edge razors to shave in the direction of hair growth. Rinse with lukewarm water and pat dry.

- If you experience irritation, apply a small amount of over-the-counter hydrocortisone cream or lotion.

Warning: If you experience significant irritation, itching, or bumps, stop! Talk to a dermatologist about removing hair with depilatories, medicated creams, or pills, or alternate hair removal methods.

Treatment of AKN

Because AKN is characterized by irritation, bumps, and keloids, the treatment is complex and there is no cure. First, you'll need to forgo the close haircuts and other practices that are irritating your skin. Then, consult a dermatologist with experience treating the condition. The form of treatment will depend on the severity of the problem. Your options include:

- *Antibiotics*. Oral medication treats any underlying infection and helps to reduce itching.
- *Topical antibiotics*. Clindamycin and erythromycin with or without benzoyl peroxide. These medications are applied once or twice daily as tolerated.
- *Retinoids*. Topical adapelene, tazarotene, or tretinoin is applied to the scalp area nightly. Dryness, irritation, and redness may develop.
- *Corticosteroids*. Topical or injected cortisone shrinks the bumps and keloids. The topical cortisones may be in the form of foams, creams, lotions, oils, or ointments.
- *Surgery*. After keloids are shrunk with cortisone, they may be surgically removed by excision or through the use of lasers.

HAIR LOSS IN MEN OF COLOR

Many men lose some if not most of their hair as they age. This is due to a combination of hereditary factors, age, and hormonal change. In men of color, however, hair thinning or loss may also occur for many of the same reasons it occurs in women of color. Men of color often abuse their hair, whether it be through the aggressive picking of a tightly coiled fro, or through the use of chemical dyes or relaxers. Depending on how they style their hair, men of color may inadvertently damage it with high-temperature hair dryers or tight cornrows or twists.

Men of color are also susceptible to developing the various forms of alopecia triggered by underlying health problems. These include *alopecia areata*, characterized by unexplained round bald spots, and *drug-induced alopecia*, which is triggered by the use of certain commonly used medications. Men undergoing cancer treatment will also lose their hair temporarily.

Hair loss in men of color typically takes the form of progressive thinning of the hair with the development of bald spots (as in "male pattern" baldness at the crown of the head) or a receding hairline. If either happens at a relatively young age, it can be difficult to deal with psychologically. But there are successful hair loss treatments available.

Handling Hair Loss

The sooner hair loss is treated, the better, so schedule a visit to a dermatologist as soon as you notice it. The physician will probably talk to you about your family history, age and hair styling habits. The treatments include:

Better Hair Care. Do you pick your hair vigorously? Or wash infrequently and skip the conditioner? You may need simply to adopt better styling practices to keep hair from breaking off or falling out. Wash hair at least once or twice a week, follow with a conditioner, and use a wide-toothed comb or natural bristle hairbrush to style. Avoid super-tight braids, twists, or ponytails, as well as heavy locks, which can pull hair out at the roots. Get trims at least once a month and try to avoid a close trim in the nape of the neck (to avoid AKN).

Corticosteroids. Topical or injected cortisone is one possible treatment for alopecia areata. Men who suffer this disease develop bald spots for a few months often followed by periods of regrowth. In many men, cortisone treatment can assist in faster regrow of the hair. The length of treatment is variable.

Hair-Loss Medications. The most promising treatments for age- or hormone-related hair loss include topical minoxidil (Rogaine Extra Strength for Men) and oral finasteride (Propecia). Your dermatologist will help determine which drug is best for your condition. Minoxidil, a liquid, is typically applied to affected areas twice a day; finasteride pills are taken once a day. It usually takes six months of use before results are noticeable. The drugs must also be used continuously; any new hair will be lost if you stop using the treatment.

Transplants. When all else fails, hair follicles can be removed from a healthy section of the head and transplanted to a bald or thinning section. Possible risks, however, include scarring and keloids.

Q&A Session

Q. *Can I use my wife's products to take care of my skin?*
A. Maybe not. Even if you may have similar skin tone, you may not have the same skin-care needs. Some men will have skin that tends to be thicker and oilier than women's. If you shave, you may have problems with dryness and bumps in that area. For those reasons, you'll benefit from products specifically designed for men and your particular skin type. Luckily for you, cosmetics companies have begun paying extra attention to the skin-care needs of men, so you should be able to find

good products. For basic skin care, wash your skin daily with a nonirritating cleanser such as those manufactured by Aveeno, Olay, or Dove; cleanse two or three times a day if your skin is oily. If you shave, follow the guidelines for shaving on page 268. Apply SPF 15 to 30 sunscreen lotion, cream, spray, or gel, or a moisturizer containing sunscreen if you tend to develop ashy skin.

Q. *How can I keep my nails looking neat?*
A. Men often neglect this area of their bodies, but poorly kept nails are more noticeable than you might think. Inspect your nails at least once a week. Clip them regularly (though not too close to the skin) and make sure they are clean underneath. If your nails are ragged-looking, shape them with an emory board and buff for shine. Moisturize your hands and nails each day with a rich moisturizer (preferably one that contains SPF 15 sunscreen) to avoid dryness and hangnails. For special occasions or simply for maintenance, splurge on a manicure to get nails filed and buffed. Consult your dermatologist if you notice a single dark streak on one nail, or other signs of poor nail health—yellow or opaque nails; white spots; thick, brittle, or twisted nails; pale nail beds; red, painful cuticles. (See chapter 11 for advice on coping with common nail-related diseases such as fungal infections.)

Q. *I have hair growing out of my nose. What do I do?*
A. This is a common problem for men. Because men have higher levels of androgens, or male hormones, more hair tends to grow and sometimes in odd places, including the nose and even the ears. To tame these hairs, keep them trimmed with a small scissor or clipper, which you can find in the drugstore. Avoid plucking hairs in these delicate areas. Make this part of your grooming ritual. You can do the same for ear-hair growth.

Q. *I'm an athlete and my wife complains about my body odor. What should I do?*
A. The best way to prevent or minimize body odor is through good hygiene. Take a shower or bath each day, especially right after you work out. Be sure to clean thoroughly under the arms, in the groin area, and between the toes with an anti-

bacterial soap. After toweling off, apply an antiperspirant/deodorant. Dry feet and sprinkle antifungal foot powders on feet and in shoes (Zeasorb AF Powder). Wear cotton clothing, including cotton socks, to absorb excess perspiration and change your clothes as necessary. Wash shirts and undershirts regularly and toss out old smelly sneakers or shoes. For excessive perspiration, your dermatologist can prescribe Drysol, a medicated antiperspirant, to decrease the sweating.

Q. *I have a lot of hair on my body, including my back. It's embarrassing. Is there anything I can do?*

A. Your excess hair growth is normal; it probably runs in your family. But that doesn't mean it's not potentially unsightly or a source of embarrassment. Some men with excessive body hair choose either to shave or to remove the hair permanently through electrolysis or laser treatments. Permanent hair-removal methods can take several treatments and may be costly. There is also a risk of discoloration in people of color. Discuss your options with a dermatologist (or electrologist) who has extensive experience with these methods to find the best solution for you.

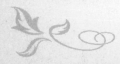

CHAPTER 16

TLC: SKIN, HAIR, AND NAIL CARE FOR CHILDREN OF COLOR

When our babies are born, their skin is soft and near perfect. But it doesn't take much time for us to notice skin problems starting to develop—dry skin, cradle cap, and eczema, to name a few. All children are susceptible to these problems, but children of color have skin that is more prone to darkening (hyperpigmentation) in response to everyday irritations and common diseases. As our kids of color grow older, they may experience dark marks for the first time owing to cuts and other injuries, as well as from putting pressure on their elbows and knees. In addition to skin concerns, their hair may begin to be affected by breakage and traction alopecia (hair loss) due to the styles—tight plaits, ponytails, cornrows—commonly worn in the Black community.

Another problem that is rampant among African-American children is a fungal scalp infection known medically as *tinea capitis*, or ringworm. Because it often looks just like dandruff, this condition often goes undiagnosed or misdiagnosed, and untreated. Tinea capitis, a contagious infection, can affect the entire family and take many frustrating weeks to cure.

As a parent, you want your child of color not only to be healthy but also to have high self-esteem. Skin, hair, and nail problems that make adults feel self-conscious can be truly devastating to a child or adolescent. That's why it's critical to keep a close eye on your youngster's skin and hair care, tend to injuries and illnesses right away, and teach your child good grooming habits as he or she grows.

YOUR CHILD'S SKIN

Newborns, small children, and teens of color may face a variety of different skin-care challenges and concerns.

Babies and Toddlers

Dry Skin. One of the first problems you might notice about your baby's skin is dryness. To prevent dry skin, only use the mildest of soaps (limit the use of soap to the diaper area—use only plain water on the remainder of the skin) and shampoos on your baby. Don't bathe him or her more than once a day. Avoid cleansers and moisturizers containing fragrances. Apply lotion or emollients such as Vaseline or Aquaphor to damp skin after bathing.

Cradle Cap. Scales and crustiness on the scalp and forehead, otherwise known as *cradle cap*, is a common problem for infants. Apply warm mineral oil to the scalp and brush very gently with a soft baby toothbrush. Then wash the hair gently. This process may be repeated every other day. It is important to avoid picking or scraping the scales off.

Eczema. If dry skin is persistent and develops into itchy, scaly, oozing, or encrusted skin, your child may have *atopic dermatitis*, or eczema. Eczema usually runs in families, especially those who have relatives with asthma, hay fever, or eczema. To tame the eczema itch, cleanse your baby or young child with only mild soaps and apply a rich lotion or emollient immediately after bathing. Avoid long baths, irritating fabrics (such as wool), and dry indoor and outdoor heat. Talk to a pediatric dermatologist if the problem is not manageable with good skin care. There are several new topical medications available for the treatment of eczema.

Rashes. A diaper rash may be resolved by simply washing a baby's bottom after each change, drying thoroughly before rediapering, and applying a protective barrier such as zinc oxide, Vaseline, or A&D ointment to the skin. Let your child go without a diaper (at home) whenever possible, and consider switching to cloth diapers. If those strategies do not work, talk to your child's doctor about prescription medications.

Older Kids and Teens

Allergic Reactions. Itchy, red skin can be caused by insect bites, exposure to poison ivy or poison oak, or nickel contained in jewelry, buckles, and buttons on pants. Besides the discomfort an allergic reaction brings about, such a reaction can make your child scratch, which will further inflame her skin. A dark mark could develop as a result. To tame the inflammation, first try to remove the offending agent, cleanse the skin completely, and apply a cool compress to soothe the area. Calamine lotion, or an over-the-counter cortisone such as Cortizone 5 or Cortaid 5 in combination with an oral antihistamine, will also help. Take your child to the doctor if an allergic reaction worsens or lasts longer than a few days.

Acne. Pimples in preteens and teens are due to the hormonal fluctuations of puberty. Although they're quite common, these bumps can be a source of extreme embarrassment and even teasing for a child. To help him or her cope, teach good skin care: cleanse skin gently twice a day with a cleanser or acne wash containing salicylic acid or a mild benzoyl peroxide; apply oil-free moisturizer if necessary; treat blemishes with benzoyl peroxide (but avoid the "maximum strength" preparations); avoid the sun; and avoid getting hair oils, gels, and hairsprays on skin. Explain how picking at pimples makes them worse and can cause dark marks to form. Take your child to the dermatologist if the acne persists or worsens.

Dark Elbows and Knees. The skin on your child's elbows and knees may turn dark because of pressure from resting his or her elbows on hard surfaces, or from kneeling and crawling. First, remind your child to avoid kneeling unless it is on soft carpeting if possible and to minimize elbow leaning. Also avoid scrubbing the areas while washing. To exfoliate and moisturize these areas, apply lotions containing glycolic or lactic acid (Eucerin Plus Lotion, Avon Intensive dry patch stick, Am-lactin Lotion). In severe cases, for older children and teens, an over-the-counter skin-bleaching cream containing 2 percent hydroquinone can help restore the skin to its natural color; just follow the manufacturer's instructions.

Scabies. If your child complains of uncontrollable itching and you notice a rash on the trunk and extremities, as well as tiny bumps and thin marks on your child's hands (between the fingers), she or he may have scabies. This condition is caused by microscopic mites that burrow under the skin, and it is spread from person to person. Your entire family can develop the rash and itching. Take your child to the dermatologist, who will prescribe a medicated cream or lotion for your child and the rest of your family members. It's important for the entire family to be treated at the same time. Wash clothing and bedding in hot water, then dry in high heat to kill the mites. Repeat the treatment after seven days to kill any eggs that may have hatched after the initial treatment.

Warts. These unsightly growths most often appear on the hands and feet. They are caused by a virus that lives in the skin cells called *human papilloma virus* (HPV). The warts are spread through skin contact. To treat a wart, first try an over-the-counter medication containing salicylic acid. The daily application of duct tape to the wart is a new treatment. If this does not work, see your dermatologist who can remove the wart with other treatments such as cutting, freezing, or burning.

Molluscum Contagiosum. These pink bumps may occur on the face, trunk, or extremities. They too are caused by a viral infection (a pox virus). Molluscum may enlarge, multiply, and become irritated. As the name implies, they are very contagious both to your child (who can quickly develop multiple growths) and to others. Although mollusca are difficult to eradicate, there are treatments including freezing and surgery. For many of our children, the mollusca will go away on their own.

Tinea Corporis. Fungal infections in children are rampant in the Black and Hispanic communities. This infectious disease is caught through direct contact between children and through the sharing of various personal objects such as combs, brushes, and hats. On the skin, tinea appears as circular flaky rings on the skin. They are often itchy and spread rapidly. It is treated with topical antifungal cream. However, any child who has tinea on the skin must be checked for scalp tinea, which is treated with an oral antifungal medication called Grifulvin V for six to eight weeks.

Daily Skin Care for Kids of Color

Teach your children or teens how to care for their skin of color now so they can maintain healthy, radiant skin for the rest of their lives:

1. Cleanse the face and body at least once a day (more if the facial skin is oily, if your child has acne or wears makeup) with a nonirritating cleanser.
2. Wash gently with the fingertips. Avoid abrasive agents such a puffs and pads.
3. Moisturize the face if necessary. Apply lotion containing an exfoliant such as glycolic acid to elbows and knees.
4. Apply SPF 15 to 30 sunscreen every day.
5. Wash hair weekly. Avoid getting hair oils or pomades on the forehead.
6. Children with oily skin or acne should pull their hair back from the face.

HAIR HELP

Your child's hair is vulnerable to many of the same problems that affect adults of color. Here are the problems to look out for.

Alopecia

The main forms of alopecia (hair loss) to look for in children are breakage and traction alopecia. In general, hair breakage tends to occur in older children and in teens. It is most likely caused by the combination of chemical relaxers and excessive heat from hair dryers, hot combs, and curling irons. If your child has breakage, you'll notice hair of various lengths, dryness, and a brittle feel to hair in the area of breakage. To heal the damage and prevent future problems such as follicular degeneration syndrome or bald spots, instruct your child or your child's hairdresser (who may be you) to take a break from harsh styling (heat, dyes, and relaxers) for a minimum of three months; wash and condition hair weekly; and apply hot-oil treatments or overnight oil treatments (see "Hair Reconstruction Regimen," page 283).

The other common source of hair loss in children of color, particularly young children, is traction alopecia. Whenever you, your child, or a stylist pulls her hair in very tight braids, braids with heavy hair ornaments, ponytails, or rollers, or if your teen wears heavy braids with extensions or weaves with extensions, hair strands can break and even come right out of the scalp. The hair root or follicle becomes inflamed from the chronic pulling or traction and small bumps, known as plait bumps (folliculitis), can develop. To stop this from causing hair loss in your child, consider a less harmful hairstyle. Or make one of the following adjustments: wearing looser braids, plaiting the hair loosely, or wearing shorter weaves and avoiding extensions or heavy hair ornaments.

Additional forms of alopecia that might affect your child or teen include alopecia areata and traumatic alopecia. See chapter 14 for descriptions of these conditions and treatment options.

Rx: Hair Reconstruction Regimen

If your child's hair is dry, brittle, and breaking, the following regimen, including products, will help to repair it (also see www.drsusantaylor.net and www.society-hilldermatology.com):

- Discontinue relaxers, texturizers, and permanent hair dyes for a six- to nine-month period.
- Trim the dead ends and even the length of your child's hair to one length all over the scalp.
- While the hair is being repaired, pull it back gently into a ponytail.
- Discontinue the application of excessive heat to hair. That means avoidance of blow dryers, hot combs, and curling irons.

In addition, institute a hair reconstruction regimen such as the following (see also websites listed above):

1. Each Friday night, saturate the hair and scalp with the hair reconstruction oil. Cover with a clear shower cap, which remains in place overnight while sleeping. Before removing the cap, apply a warm towel over the cap for ten minutes or sit under a hood dryer for ten minutes.
2. Remove the cap and wash hair thoroughly with the oil-removing shampoo and rinse.
3. Lather up with the conditioning shampoo and leave on for two minutes.
4. Rinse thoroughly and then apply the deep conditioner for fifteen minutes. Your child may sit under a hooded dryer during this period of time or wrap a warm towel around the head.

5. Rinse, comb with a wide-tooth comb, and gently dry the hair (either air-dry or sit under a hooded dryer).

6. Throughout the week, apply the hair repair cream to the ends of the hair.

7. For itching and flaking of the scalp, throughout the week apply a small amount of the hair reconstruction oil directly onto the scalp.

8. At bedtime, have your child wear a satin scarf or cap so that the hair does not get caught on the pillow case and break overnight.

Strict adherence to this regime for the next six to nine months will result in healthier, softer, and stronger hair.

Head Lice

Your child may come home from school with more than new ideas in her head. Tiny insects, known as lice, can spread from child to child through touch or the sharing of combs, brushes, or hats. The lice will make your child's scalp itch. To get rid of the critters, use a medicated shampoo (Rid or Nix), which needs to be left on the scalp as directed (it is important to follow the directions exactly as written). Also, wash all bedding and clothes in hot water, then dry in high heat. Finally, the removal of the eggs (called nits) is crutial to eradicating the infestation. Special narrow-tooth combs are available to remove the nits. It's not necessary to cut or shave the child's hair to eradicate the infection.

Tinea Capitis (Ringworm)

This prevalent condition is caused by a fungus. It is often mistaken for dandruff because the symptoms are similar: itching, scaling, inflammation. You might also notice red bumps or pus bumps on the scalp. In the most severe cases, your child might even suffer hair loss and a pus-filled swelling of the scalp called a *kerion*. If you even suspect this problem, see your doctor immediately. A delay could result in prolonged discomfort for your child and permanent hair loss. The treatment for tinea capitis is prescription antifungal medication, which needs to be taken for as long as six or eight weeks. You'll also need to make sure other family members, especially siblings, have not caught the condition since it is spread through contact and the sharing of brushes, combs, and hats.

Hair Products and Early Puberty—Is There a Link?

There have been a few reports in medical literature about young girls undergoing premature puberty (pubic hair, breast development before age twelve) owing to the use of hair/scalp products that contain "estrogen complex." One such product is B&B Supergro. It is thought that the estrogen in the product is absorbed into the system, causing breast and pubic hair development.

To prevent this from happening to your child, the first thing that you should do is check the labels of all of the hair-care products that your child uses. If you do find in the list of ingredients either estrogens or hormones, discontinue use immediately. Then inform your child's pediatrician so that your child may be evaluated.

Relaxers in Kids

You may wonder when it is safe to bring your daughter to the hair salon for her first hair relaxer. I do not recommend the use of hair relaxers in young children. As a dermatologist, I see so much hair loss in young adult women, and often we do not know the cause. Some dermatologists think that this hair loss may be related to relaxer use. For that reason, I think you should wait until your child is a teen before considering her first relaxer.

NAIL CARE

Your child's nails are also vulnerable to problems. The following are problems to look out for:

Ingrown Toenails

If your child has pain and redness in the toe, particularly the big toe, he or she may have an ingrown toenail. This is often caused by wearing too-tight socks or shoes. To cure it, first try an over-the-counter ingrown toenail treatment. If that does not work, you may need to take your child to the doctor for antibiotic treatment and possible removal of the ingrown portion of the nail.

Nail Biting

Many young and older children bite their nails, a bad habit that often starts as a way to cope with stress. Nail biting not only makes the nails and hands look unkempt but it also increases the likelihood that your child will pick up and spread germs. Talk to your child about the nail biting. To discourage nail biting, you may want to teach her or him good nail care: use mild soaps to cleanse hands and under the nails; moisturize with creamy lotions; clip nails regularly, and file them in one direction.

Nail Fungus

Although nail infections are less common in children than in adults, they can occur. A child who spends a lot of time at public swimming pools or in a sports team locker room may pick up a fungal infection in the nails or toenails. The signs are white or yellow spots on nails, and nails that turn a different color (yellow, green, brown, black) or thicken. In the worst case, an infected nail will separate from the nail bed. Depending upon your child's age, the treatment is either a topical antifungal nair polish or an oral antifungal medication. If a nail is very painful, take your child to the doctor, who can remove it in order for a new, healthy one to grow.

Index

Page numbers in italics refer to illustrations.

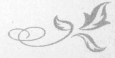